Francislene Lopes Menezes
Suzinara B. S. de Lima
Teresinha Heck Weiller

Nurses' work with women in the Family Health Strategy

Francislene Lopes Menezes
Suzinara B. S. de Lima
Teresinha Heck Weiller

Nurses' work with women in the Family Health Strategy

Nurses' work with women

ScienciaScripts

Imprint

Cover image: www.ingimage.com

This book is a translation from the original published under ISBN 978-613-9-70426-2.

Publisher:
Sciencia Scripts
is a trademark of
Dodo Books Indian Ocean Ltd. and OmniScriptum S.R.L publishing group

120 High Road, East Finchley, London, N2 9ED, United Kingdom
Str. Armeneasca 28/1, office 1, Chisinau MD-2012, Republic of Moldova, Europe
Printed at: see last page
ISBN: 978-620-8-21165-3

CONTENTS

CHAPTER 1

INTRODUCTION

Historically, the modern perception of primary health care emerged in the UK in 1920 in the Dawnson report, which advocated organising the health service system into three levels: primary and secondary health care centres and teaching hospitals. This document describes the functions of each level of care and the relationships that should exist between them. This proposal forms the basis for the regionalisation of health services organised on a population basis, and has inspired the organisation of health systems in several countries around the world (MENDES, 2002).

Primary health care (PHC) in Brazil has come a long way before reaching its contemporary status. It was introduced in different countries as a strategy for organising health care aimed at meeting most of a population's health needs in a regionalised, continuous and systematised way, involving preventive and curative actions, as well as care for individuals and communities (MATTA; MOROSINI, 2008).

At the beginning of the 20th century in Brazil, health centres maintained the division between curative and preventive actions, were organised on a population basis and worked with health education. From the 1940s onwards, the Special Public Health Service (SESP) was created, which carried out curative and preventive actions, albeit restricted to infectious and deficiency diseases. This experience, initially limited to economically important areas such as rubber extraction, was extended during the 1950s and 1960s to other regions of the country. From the 1960s to the mid-1980s, the medical-privatist model was implemented (MENDES, 2002).

This model began during Brazil's industrialisation period to meet the health needs of workers, with the aim of preventing the working class from falling ill and consequently avoiding losses in the economic sector. It was clinic-centred, focused on meeting spontaneous demand and based on specialised procedures and services. This model ended up being criticised because there was unequal access, low resolution and productivity of resources, excessive centralisation and no interaction between the different types of services.

With the politics of the 1980s, the financial crisis and the redemocratisation movement, the country stimulated a process that sought to transform the old ways of offering health services to the population into a model based on general doctrinal principles - such as universality, integrality and equity - which became a fundamental right of the Brazilian people in the area of health. The health reform movement, whose efforts focused on more general health policy issues, culminated in the 8th National Health Conference (8ª), which was instrumental in the construction of the Constitution promulgated in 1988 and the creation of the Unified Health System (SUS), organised into principles and guidelines that defined PHC as the guiding and articulating guideline for transforming the current health care model (BRASIL, 201 la). The principles that underpin the SUS are universality, equity and comprehensive health services, and its organisational principles are decentralisation, regionalisation and hierarchisation of the network, as well as social participation (BRASIL, 1990a).

In Brazil, the Family Health Strategy (ESF) is the main strategy for implementing and organising PHC. The Family Health Programme (PSF) was created in 1994 and presented in the first ministerial document as a programme. It was then considered a strategy for reorienting the care model in accordance with the principles of the SUS. Contrary to the idea held about most programmes at central level, the PSF is not a vertical intervention that runs parallel to the activities of the health services: it is a strategy that makes integration possible and promotes the organisation of these activities in a defined territory (BRASIL, 2001a).

The work in the ESF unit must be interdisciplinary and team-based, integrating technical areas and professionals from different backgrounds, valuing diverse knowledge and practices with a view to a comprehensive and resolutive approach, enabling the creation of bonds of trust with ethics, commitment and respect (BRASIL, 2006a).

For Mendes-Gonçalves (1994), work is determined by a need or want; it is the means of subsistence for the satisfaction of material and non-material needs and also the enabler of free creation. It is understood as a human activity carried out by a group of people who dedicate themselves to it and thus reproduce a human existence.

When work is related to health, the result is the development of an intersessional space between the user and the health worker, where the health worker meets the user's needs, often seen as a lack of health or a more autonomous way of travelling in the world. The purpose of health work is to provide individual or collective care, resulting in the healing and health of the citizen. Therefore, health work is produced at the exact moment of consumption, which is why it is so dynamic (MERHY, 2007).

Nursing work is understood as a social practice and is articulated with other health practices, such as health education, the production of medicines and equipment, among others. In addition, it incorporates the provision of health services in the tertiary sector, not producing goods to be stockpiled and traded, but services to be consumed at the point of care, be it individual, group or collective. It differs from other jobs in the same tertiary service sector in that it deals with a human object, such as users, who bring demands associated with the health-disease process, demonstrated as health needs or problems (FELLI; PEDUZZI, 2005).

Among the various fields of work for nurses, two areas stand out: public health work and hospital care. The nurse who works in the ESF Unit is a key member of the basic multidisciplinary team and must carry out nursing consultations, order complementary tests, transcribe/prescribe medication in accordance with protocols established by the Ministry of Health (MS) and legal provisions of the profession, work in the planning, management, coordination, execution and evaluation of the Unit, considering the real needs of the population. In addition, they are responsible for providing comprehensive care for children, adolescents, women, adults and the elderly; they must combine clinical work with collective health practice; carry out activities corresponding to the priority areas for intervention in basic care, defined in the Basic Care Operational Standard; supervise and train Community Health Workers (CHWs) and nursing assistants, with a view to improving their performance; provide direct nursing care in clinical urgencies and emergencies, making referrals for continuity of care (BRASIL, 2002a).

In addition to these various duties of the profession, carrying out actions recommended by the Ministry of Health's programmes and adapting these programmes to the reality of the community are also the nurse's obligations. Women's Health programmes and policies are one of the broadest areas of activity within the ESF unit.

According to the Ministry of Health, nurses are responsible for women's health: acting directly in contraceptive care with educational activities, counselling and clinical activities, as well as providing care for marital infertility with pregnancy-related counselling (BRASIL, 2002b). According to the guidelines in the Ministry of Health's Prenatal and Puerperium Manual (BRASIL, 2006b), nurses are also responsible for carrying out educational activities for women and their families; carrying out low-risk prenatal consultations; requesting routine tests and guiding treatment according to the service protocol; referring pregnant women identified as being at risk to the doctor; carrying out activities with pregnant women's groups, waiting room groups; carrying out home visits; when appropriate, providing the pregnant woman's card duly updated at each consultation and carrying out the cytopathological examination.

In an attempt to improve women's health care, over the years the Ministry of Health has advocated various policies and programmes that have defined activities for women's health. In 1984, the Ministry of Health drew up the Comprehensive Women's Health Care Programme (PAISM), signalling a new and differentiated approach to women's health. This programme was driven by the principles of Health Reform, integrated into the search for the principles of decentralisation, regionalisation of services, equity in care and community participation in order to transform and value women's health care, essentially seeking care at all stages of women's lives (BRASIL, 2011b).

The Comprehensive Women's Health Care Programme preceded a number of women's policies, for example, in June 2000, the Ministry of Health set up the Prenatal and Birth Humanisation Programme (PHPN) to ensure the humanisation of services, access and quality of prenatal care, childbirth care, postpartum care and neonatal care (BRASIL, 2013a).

In 2004, the National Policy for Comprehensive Women's Health Care -

Principles and Guidelines was presented, which recalls the situation of women's lives and health, as well as new focuses in women's care, with the aim of promoting improvements in the living conditions and health of Brazilian women, by guaranteeing legally constituted rights and expanding access to means and services for health promotion, prevention, care and recovery throughout Brazil; reduce female morbidity and mortality in the country, especially from preventable causes, in all life cycles and in the various population groups, without discrimination of any kind. This government strategy also seeks to expand, qualify and humanise women's health care within the SUS health services. In addition, it expands the actions in its action plans to groups that have historically been forgotten by public policies, in terms of their specificities and needs, including lesbian, bisexual and climacteric women, women from the countryside and the forest, Indians, black quilombolas, women who experience transsexuality, women in prison, women with disabilities, women living on the streets and gypsies (BRASIL, 2009a).

In this dimension, the ESF unit seeks to offer the consolidation of these new profiles of the women's health situation in Brazil, based on the reorganisation/change in the care model for women's care, bringing health services and professionals closer to families and communities, programming and articulating actions based on local needs (CUNHA et al, 2011).

When carrying out the literature review, with the aim of analysing the nurse's work process in the ESF Units, we sought to find out about the research carried out on this subject. The review was carried out using the Nursing Database (BDENF), the *Scientific Electronic Library Online (Scielo*) and the Latin American and Caribbean Literature on Health Sciences (LILACS), using the descriptors: "nursing", "Family Health Programme" and "work".

Thus, a total of 9 articles made up the corpus of analysis, i.e. 1 in LILACS, 6 in BDENF and 2 in *Scielo.* The following inclusion criteria were applied: productions available free of charge *online* in their entirety; in Portuguese, English and Spanish and with a time frame of 2000-2012. Texts that were not freely available *online,* did not deal specifically with the topic and were duplicated were excluded from the analysis.

In the light of the scientific literature, it can be seen that the work of nurses in basic health services is very important, and that they are a central part of the functioning of the units - a situation that generates an accumulation of responsibilities, in addition to what is recommended by the concept of the Family Health Strategy. It can be seen that there is little published research on this subject. This highlights the pertinence of further studies into nurses' work, in order to reflect on work organisation, professional qualification and performance and, above all, the provision of a quality service for all users.

My initial interest in the subject of nursing work with women is justified as a consequence of my academic career, after taking the Specialisation Course in Public Health Organisation Management at the Federal University of Santa Maria. The conclusion of the course, in the form of an article, entitled "Puerperal Depression within the Public Health Network", dealt with programmes and actions aimed at caring for women within the public health system. This approach contributed to reflections and concerns about the work carried out by nurses in Basic Health Units with women, bearing in mind that their health is a priority in the context of the federal management of the SUS, proposing targets to ensure access to essential services at all stages of the life cycle.

In addition, while taking part in the activities of the "Nursing and Health Management" Group, linked to the "Work, Health, Education and Nursing" Research Group, occasions arose for discussions and reflections on the day-to-day work in health institutions, as this is a need to improve the quality of care provided.

In this sense, the **research question is:** How do nurses work with women in the ESF units in the municipality of Santa Maria/RS? And the object of study: the work of nurses with women in ESF units.

This question led to the following objectives:

General objective:

- To get to know the work of nurses with women in the Family Health Strategy Units (ESF) in the municipality of Santa Maria/RS, by analysing interviews conducted with these professionals.

Specific objectives:

- To identify the facilities and difficulties of nurses' work with women in the ESF units of Santa Maria/RS;

- To identify the strategies used by nurses when working with women in the ESF units of Santa Maria/RS;

This research is relevant because it suggests that nurses, staff and health managers should reflect on the work being done in ESF units, taking into account what is recommended in the SUS. In this way, actions can be developed that are consistent with serving women in the ESF units, qualifying the know-how and providing visibility, autonomy and efficiency to the work.

CHAPTER 2
LITERATURE REVIEW

2.1 The Unified Health System and Women's Health

The Unified Health System (SUS) was created in 1988 by the Brazilian Constitution to offer universal health care and promote the health of the entire population. The system is a unique social project that materialises through actions to promote, prevent and assist the health of Brazilians. Before its creation, health care was subdivided according to the social classes of users: those who could afford private health services, those who had the right to public health because they were insured by the social security system (salaried workers) and those who had no rights at all. The establishment of the SUS unified the system, since before 1988 health was the responsibility of several ministries, and decentralised its management. It ceased to be the exclusive responsibility of the Federal Executive Branch and began to be administered by states and municipalities.

According to the Ministry of Health, the SUS has more than 6,500 accredited hospitals, 45,000 primary care units and 30,300 Family Health Teams. The system carries out 2.8 billion annual outpatient procedures, 19,000 transplants, 236,000 heart surgeries, 9.7 million chemotherapy and radiotherapy procedures and 11 million hospitalisations. Among the SUS's most recognised actions are the creation of the Mobile Emergency Care Service (SAMU), the National Policies for Integral Attention to Women's Health, Humanisation of the SUS and Workers' Health, as well as mass vaccination programmes for children and the elderly throughout the country and transplants carried out by the public network (BRASIL, 2009b).

In 1994, in an attempt to reorganise the care model, the ESF unit was created, which became another gateway for the population into the health system and was considered a mechanism for reorganising Primary Health Care (PHC) in the country.

According to the Ministry of Health, the ESF is a set of individual and collective actions carried out to promote health and prevent illnesses, as well as to provide care for health problems. The actions produced in this strategy are the privileged moment to provide resolutive actions, which fully and more comprehensively address the needs beyond health care (BRASIL, 2012a).

The nurse's role in the ESF unit is fundamental for planning, executing and evaluating health programming, as well as health surveillance actions. They work individually or at the interface with multi-professional teams when drawing up, implementing and evaluating therapeutic health plans (BRASIL, 2011a). It is up to nurses to provide equal care to their population, while maintaining the individuality of each person, helping to prevent illness, promote health and improve quality of life. However, one of the points of attention is the health of women, who are involved in their social, cultural and economic environment.

To set up the ESF unit, the Ministry of Health uses policies and some assistance programmes that take into account the preferred demands of the community linked to the basic health unit and allow public policies to become effective.

National policies for women's health care were introduced in the first decades of the 20th century, determining the demands related to pregnancy and childbirth. In the 1930s, 1950s and 1970s, maternal and child programmes had a restricted view of women, based on their biological specificity and their social role as mothers and domestic workers, responsible for raising, educating and caring for the health of their children and other family members (BRASIL, 2011b).

In 1994, the Ministry of Health drew up the National Comprehensive Care Policy (PAISM), which has the programme "Comprehensive Care for Women's Health: bases for programmatic action". The PAISM proposes that care be provided at all stages of life, gynaecological clinic, reproduction (reproductive planning, pregnancy, childbirth and the puerperium), as well as in cases of chronic or acute illness. It recognises care as medical care and the care of the entire health team, prioritising educational practices that include women's critical capacity and autonomy (BRASIL,
2013b). The programme brings together the SUS principles of decentralisation, hierarchisation and regionalisation of services, as well as comprehensive and equitable

care, including educational, preventive, diagnostic, treatment and recovery actions (BRASIL, 2011b).

The construction of the SUS has had a strong influence on the implementation of PAISM. The SUS has been implemented on the basis of the principles and guidelines contained in the basic legislation: the 1988 Constitution, Law No. 8.080 and Law No. 8.142, the Basic Operational Standards (NOB) and the Operational Standards for Health Care (NOAS), published by the Ministry of Health (BRASIL, 2011b).

The Operational Standard for Health Care (NOAS 2001) aims to expand the responsibilities of municipalities in primary care, creating mechanisms to strengthen the management of the SUS, updating the qualification criteria for states and municipalities (BRASIL, 2011b). Among the Primary Health Care responsibilities to be carried out are women's health actions, aimed at prevention, family planning and prenatal care.

In 2004, the National Pact for the Reduction of Maternal and Neonatal Mortality was launched, which promotes the improvement of obstetric and neonatal care through the mobilisation and participation of federal, state and municipal managers and organised civil society - universities, medical societies and non-governmental organisations (NGOs) - in a broad social dialogue that aims, among other things, to promote and monitor the actions carried out by the Ministry of Health to reduce maternal and neonatal mortality. This initiative was awarded by the United Nations (UN) as a model of social mobilisation and dialogue for the promotion of the Millennium Development Goals (MDGs), even before 2015 (BRASIL, 2009a).

In 2005, the National Policy on Sexual Rights and Reproductive Rights was launched. This was responsible for encouraging the adoption of good practices in obstetric and neonatal care, based on scientific evidence in almost 500 maternity reference centres in the 27 federal units, and the qualification of care for obstetric urgencies/emergencies in maternity hospitals and SAMU (BRASIL, 2009a).

Women's health is a priority in the context of the federal management of the SUS, since women make up the majority of the Brazilian population (50.77%) and are the main users of the SUS. They seek care for themselves, but especially for their children, partners and other family members (BRASIL, 201 lb).

In 2011, a national programme called Rede Cegonha (Stork Network) was created with the aim of providing adequate, safe and humanised care, from the confirmation of pregnancy, through prenatal care, childbirth and the puerperium, to the first two years of the child's life (BRASIL, 2011c). The Stork Network is a strategy set up by the Ministry of Health and operationalised by the SUS. This initiative is based on humanisation and care for women, newborns and children. By 2014, it aims to qualify care in order to expand and improve conditions for the birth of all Brazilians, with an emphasis on humanisation and safety (BRASIL, 2011c). The aim of this programme is to implement a pioneering model of care for women's and children's health, focusing on care during labour and birth and child development up to the age of two. By setting up and organising a Maternal and Child Health Care Network, the aim is to reduce maternal and child mortality rates, with a focus on the neonatal aspect (BRASIL, 2013c).

2.2 The Health Work Process

Recent years have seen considerable changes in various sectors of society. These include the labour market, politics, with the progressive and effective participation of women; in health, this participation is also intense, since women make up the majority of the world's elderly population and are becoming mothers at an increasingly younger age. Consequently, all of this requires changes in health services in terms of the structure and production processes of actions.

Human beings' understanding of the meaning of work begins at an early age; they soon learn that if something is done for a specific purpose, transformation, consideration, respect and appreciation are achieved. Tavares (2011) says that the correct evolutionary cycle of life would be: being born, growing up, working, reproducing and dying. Evolution is part of life, so human beings see work as a way of meeting their needs, of achieving fulfilment, of participating and getting something back for their efforts.

For Mendes-Gonçalves (1994), work is understood as a human activity carried out by a group of people who dedicate themselves to it and thus reproduce a human existence. Work is determined by a need or want and is the means of subsistence for satisfying material and non-material needs. In health, in a more operational concept, these needs are almost always associated with the assistance and care provided.

According to Pires (2008), health work is essential to human life, being in the sphere of non-material production and being completed in the act of its realisation. The provision of this service, in other words, the act of care itself, involves the work of different professionals with special knowledge and techniques to assist individuals or groups. Peduzzi (1998, p. 48) states that the involvement of these different professionals, each carrying out their own specialised activities, constitute processes that complement each other, expanding the possibilities of "recognising and attending to the health needs of users, in terms of efficiency and effectiveness".

According to Campos (2006), the health work process has undergone notable transformations, especially with industrialisation and the incorporation of countless scientific advances and discoveries in order to preserve life.

The implementation of the ESF units was an important resource for the rise of the Brazilian healthcare model. It established client registration, multi-professional teamwork and the participation of the population - in a logic that breaks with the professional-centred model and strives to get closer to the life of the community. Its work process enables commitment and co-responsibility between the team and the user, as well as the articulation between the different types of knowledge of the professional organisations that make up this care model (BRASIL, 2001b).

Nursing, as a component of the FHS unit's work process, is responsible for contributing to the inclusion of new technologies and new knowledge in the work process of these teams. Its institutionalisation as part of the health work process only became evident as a profession in the mid-19th century in England with Florence Nightingale. It is structured from a capitalist production point of view and, intrinsically, is evidenced by the division of labour. Its institutionalisation is accompanied by two other striking aspects: discipline and hierarchy (PEDUZZI; ANSELMI, 2002).

According to Rocha and Almeida (2000), nursing is understood as a social practice, that is, as a part of health work that establishes social relations in the production of services. It is placed in the world of work and in health work specifically, as part of collective work and is influenced by it.

Nursing work, as an instrument of the health work process, is subdivided into various dimensions, such as care/assistance, administration/management, research and teaching, and political participation. Among these, caring and managing are the processes most evident in nurses' work, whether in primary care or hospital settings (SANNA, 2007).

According to Merhy (2007), in health work, professionals have the following tools: soft technologies - which include the types of approach used by health professionals in "intersection spaces", such as welcoming, linking, making people accountable and others; soft-hard technologies - made up of the structured knowledge of different professionals and categories - and hard technologies, which are diagnostic aids, medical-hospital materials, etc. For this author, the care model developed in a given health system is expressed through the use and management of these technologies. These enable the creation of spaces for co-operation and the exchange of knowledge between different health professionals, allowing for the expansion of interdisciplinary, articulated and collective work within the team itself, especially with a view to exchanging the knowledge and experiences of each individual involved in the process of providing health care to the population.

Pinheiro (2011) points out that, in practice, the nurse who works in the ESF unit is faced with unexpected realities and needs to develop skills to deal with the complexity of the work process in order to help solve a variety of problems. Therefore, the issues presented by the demands go beyond the disease and require different tools for decision-making. In the ESF, the way in which work processes operate to encourage healthy living must be aligned with the possibility of tackling inequalities in people's living conditions, including access to services and goods that help to ensure a good quality of life.

Passos (2011) points out that the role of the nurse in the ESF unit is very broad, opening up a range of possibilities for organising their work in multiple ways, thus being able to address the issues of a new pro-status health model.

2.3 The Family Health Strategy and the Nurse

The Family Health Programme (PSF) began when the Ministry of Health formulated the Community Health Agents Programme (PACS) in 1991, with the aim of helping to reduce infant and maternal mortality, especially in the North and Northeast regions of Brazil, by extending health service coverage to the poorest and most deprived areas. Based on the experience accumulated in Ceará with PACS, the Ministry of Health realised the importance of agents in basic health services in the state and began to focus on the family as the unit of health programme action, no longer highlighting only the individual, but introducing the notion of coverage by family. In this way, the PSF was conceived from a meeting held on 27 and 28 December 1993 in Brasilia, DF, on the subject of "Family Health", convened by the office of Health Minister Henrique Santillo, with the support of the United Nations Children's Fund (UNICEF). The meeting was based on the discussion of a new proposal based on the success of PACS and the need to integrate new professionals, so that the agents would not work in isolation. In January 1994, the first Family Health teams were formed, integrating and extending the work of community health workers (ROSA; LABATE, 2005).

The Ministry of Health proposed the Family Health Programme strategy as a way of reorganising the production of health care in primary care, which would be a new way of doing health. The aim of developing this strategy was to reorganise health care practice on new bases and criteria, replacing the traditional model of care, which is oriented towards curing diseases and centred on the hospital. "This new strategy requires health professionals to have a broader understanding of the health-disease process and, above all, modes of intervention that go beyond curative practice" (FRANCO; MERHY, 2003, p. 28).

Currently, the PSF is defined as the Family Health Strategy (ESF), rather than a programme, since the term programme refers to an activity that begins, develops and ends. The ESF is a strategy for reorganising primary care and does not foresee a timeframe for completing this reorganisation (COSTA; TRINDADE; PEREIRA, 2010). It reaffirms and incorporates the basic principles of the SUS: universalisation, decentralisation, comprehensiveness and popular participation. It is structured on the basis of a public health unit, with a multi-professional and interdisciplinary team, which assumes responsibility for a specific population linked to it, where it carries out actions to promote health and prevent, treat and rehabilitate illnesses (BRASIL, 2001a).

The ESF has shown positive results, i.e. it has improved maternal and child health, reduced infant mortality, increased access to prenatal care, family planning and the prevention of complications from chronic diseases (BRASIL, 2008). It acts at all stages of human development and has some specific strategic areas, limited by the Ministry of Health, to act throughout the national territory, including: the elimination of child malnutrition, control of hypertension, women's health, the health of the elderly, children's health, oral health and health promotion (BRASIL, 2006a).

Family health teams are made up of a doctor, a nurse, a nursing assistant or technician and up to 12 community health workers. Each team is responsible for the situation in a given territory and carries out promotion, prevention, diagnosis, treatment and rehabilitation actions through home visits, educational work and visits to basic health units.

According to the National Primary Care Policy - Ordinance 648/2006 - (BRASIL, 2006a), which deals with the duties of the professionals who make up the Family Health Team, the specific duties of the Family Health nurse are: to carry out nursing consultations; to plan, manage, coordinate and evaluate the actions carried out by the CHAs; to supervise, coordinate and carry out continuing education activities for the CHAs and the nursing team; to participate in the management of the supplies necessary for the proper functioning of the Basic Health Unit (BRASIL, 2006a).

Nurses have gained ground in primary care because of their prominence in consolidating the ESF, but there are still obstacles to the work process within the team, making it a challenge for them to reconcile their demands. In this sense, the Primary Care actions that should be carried out by the Family Health team, through interdisciplinary work, are in practice carried out individually, with the nurse taking on most of the responsibilities, including managing the Health Unit (FREITAS; NUNES, 2010). Interdisciplinary and teamwork is one of the foundations of Primary Care and is also one of the characteristics of the Family Health team's work process (BRASIL, 2006a).

The interdisciplinary team is a privileged space for establishing more egalitarian relationships between those involved, since it presumes the construction of other ways of experiencing the management and organisation of health work, with everyone participating in the planning, execution and overall evaluation of care. In the context of health work, interdisciplinarity is a process under construction in which the various disciplines/professionals are involved in pursuit of a common goal - comprehensive care for service users. In this process, some components are indispensable: authentic communication, dialogue, respect and recognition of the knowledge and work of each professional and the possibility of participation in decision-making (MATTOS; PIRES; CAMPOS, 2009). This interdisciplinary team is made up of a general practitioner, a nurse, a nursing technician, community health workers and a dentist. The nurse is largely responsible for coordinating and supervising the work of this team, especially the nursing technician and the community health worker.

One of the most complex and comprehensive aspects of the FHS is women's health care. Therefore, nurses must be able to work in various areas of women's health, with a view to assisting them at all stages of their development, making it an essential tool for improving health indicators (SALMERON; FUCITALO, 2008). Prenatal care, family planning, prevention of cervical cancer, prevention of dental problems and oral diseases, especially tooth decay and gum disease, are the main activities of this type of care.

The World Health Organisation (WHO) estimates that, due to the less interventionist characteristics of their care, nurses are the least expensive professionals and provide the most affective actions to achieve safe motherhood, reduce morbidity and mortality and the costs of caring for women in both the pregnancy and puerperal cycles. The Brazilian government has endeavoured to promote the training of human resources, including obstetric nurses, with the aim of increasing their numbers and reversing the country's situation through the qualification of the staff who care for women. The importance of nursing work in primary care is recognised, and nurses play a fundamental role in essential public health functions. This has been recognised by both managers and the general population (CAGNIN, 2008).

2.4 The Nurses' Work Process in Family Health Strategy Units

The work process in primary health care is strongly linked to living labour, the nature and content of the activity, technical and scientific quality, motivation and the worker's commitment to the outcome of their work (FACCHINI et al., 2006).

Nursing competently and responsibly integrates the processes associated with health, acts in the protection and recovery of sick people, endeavours to satisfy the health needs of the population, and aims to promote health and quality of life (RAMOS et al., 2009).

Given the importance of studying the work process, the aim was to identify the profile of scientific production and how the work process of nurses in FHS units is going. To this end, in March 2013, a search was carried out in the databases Nursing Database (BDENF), *Scientific Electronic Library Online (Scielo*) and Latin American and Caribbean Literature in Health Sciences (LILACS). The inclusion criteria for the articles selected for this review were: articles available *online* in their entirety free of charge; in Portuguese, English and Spanish and with the time frame 2000-2012. The exclusion criteria were: texts that were not freely available *online,* did not deal specifically with the subject and were duplicated. The words "nursing", "Family Health Programme" and "work" were used as descriptors, associated with the Boolean operator "and", as a way of capturing a comprehensive number of publications.

Three publications were found in LILACS, 91 in BDENF and 14 *in Scielo*, totalling 108 articles. After selecting the publications, a total of 9 articles made up the *corpus* of analysis, i.e. 1 in LILACS, 6 in BDENF and 2 in *Scielo*. The data was organised using a synoptic table (Chart 1), which enabled the profile of the scientific productions to be outlined.

N°	Authors	Year	Journal	Title	Aim of the study	Results
1.	Emiko Yoshikawa Egry, Rosa Maria Godoy Serpa da Fonseca	2000	Journal of the School of Nursing ofUSP	The family, home visits and nursing: revisiting the health nursing work process collective.	Discuss the conceptual issues underlying the family and home visits, contextualised in the context of health production in Brazil, h ighlighting the The Family Care Programme and the Theory of Practical Nu rsing Interventionin Collective Health.	It is opportune for public health nursing to use the Home Visit tool to carry out relevant to Family Health Programme (PSF). This perspective will be realised when the practice is competently carried out by current workers in the field of public health nursing, at the same time that the institutions trainers value and include the knowledge necessary for this practice in their study programmes.
2.	Dalvani Marques, Eliete Maria Silva	2004	Brazilian Journal of Nursing	Nursing and the He alth Programme Family: a par tnership success?	Analysing nu rsing work Family Health Programme (PSF).	The nurse's work is more foc used on the unit and on the patients. procedures The nurse's role is essentially managerial and she still works on the basis of the demand that arrives at the units and what the CHAs identify.
3.	Regina Célia Ermel, Lislaine Aparecida Fracolli	2006	Journal of the School of Nursing ofUSP	The work of nurses in the Family Health Programme in Marília/SP.	Characterising the nurse's work process in the PSF, identifying its object, purpose, means and instruments.	Nurses take the individual body as the object of their work , the purpose of which is to intervene in the wear and tear profiles of social groups and operate in this way. working with instruments traditional public health, such as the Consultade Nursing and Home Visits. The analysis of the data also showed that the nurses at the PSF in Marília/SP,

						when exercising their practice, they reiterate the logic of clinical, individual, curative practice and act on the basis of reference to the multicausality theory of the health process-disease.
4.	Viviane Camargo Santos, Cássia Baldini Soares, Célia Maria Sivalli Campos	2007	Journal of the School of Nursing ofUSP	Relationship work-health of PSF nurses in the municipality of São Paulo.	You'll understand characteristics of the work of nurses and the relationship between the processes of empowerment and attrition that are expressed in them.	The work is almost always the result of tension between social and health reality found in the territories and the imposition of targets that do not address the problems brought by the population. The organisation of work puts workers in front of the challenge of meeting targets, taking part in meetings and, at the same time, dealing with unforeseen events, ranging from demands for answers to problems that are not solved. extrapolate programmes planned for users, to administrative demands, which are often go beyond the duties previously stipulated for workers.
5.	Jesanne Barguil Brasileiro Rocha, Regina Célia Gollner Zeitoune	2007	UERJ Nursing Journal	Profiles Programme nurses Health Family: a need to discuss professional practice	You will analyse characteristics of nurses who working in the Family Health Programme (PSF) in Floriano (PI) in 2006, and discuss the implications for professional practice.	They showed that the majority are over 30 years old, have a temporary contract with the town hall, and have double employment . employment, acts in parallel in the teaching and/or hospital care; 33.3 per cent of professionals have specialised in Public Health and most of them have been

						working in the PSF for more than three years. They identified the need technical and scientific training to work in the PSF and decentralisation of postgraduate courses in especially in the area of Family Health. It is suggested that the way professionals are hired be reviewed.
6.	Raquel Gusmão Oliveira, Sônia Silva Marcon	2007	Journal of the School of Nursing ofUSP	Working with families in the Health Programme Family nurse practice in Maringá-Paraná	Get to know the practice of working with families nurses working in the PSF in Maringá, Paraná.	Health education and reception are still marked by the traditional, curative and individual model of care. Nurses believe they are looking after the family, even though when their work process does not differ from the one adopted to assist the individual, leading them to consider that what is happening is assistance to the individual. individuals who have family members and not family care as a unit of care.
7.	Maria Denise Schimith, Maria Alice Diasda Silva Lima	2009	UERJ Nursing Journal	The Nurse in the Healthcare Team Family: study case.	To analyse the work process of nurses in a family health team.	The nurse's work object in the teamfia collective need of users, despite wanting to carry out clinical actions and get closer to the population . nurse primarily carries out administrative and collective education; coordinating supervises activities carried out by community health workers.
8.	Cinara da	2009	Journal of	Pr	To describe the profile	

	Silva Ramos, Rita Maria Heck, Teila Ceolin, Alitéia Santiago Dilélio, Luiz Augusto Facchini		Science, Care and Health	ofile nurse working in the Strategy He alth Family	of nurses working in the Family Health Strategy in six municipalities in the southern region of Rio Grande do Sul.	The the need for nurses to have a diagnosis of the place where they work, in order to plan health actions, with the participation of community, taking into account the local reality and culture, so as to enable the reorganisation of health practices.
9.	Jennyesle Lima Castro de Santiago, Juliana Macêdo de Medeiros, Fernanda M. F. Castelo Branco, Christiane Lopes Xavier, Iluska Borges Dias, Claudete Ferreira de Souza Monteiro	2011	Research Journal: Care is Fundamental Online	The nursing work process in supervision.	Describe the work process of nurses supervising the Family Health Teams; to identify the challenges experienced by supervisors in the process of supervising Family Health Teams and to discuss the possibilities of new working practices that contribute to implementation of the model centred on prevention and health promotion.	Supervisors emphasised importance of planning with the teams, however emphasised work overload related to solving the administrative problems of the Basic Health Unit as a challenge aser overcome.

Chart 1- Characteristics of studies on the nursing work process, according to the authors, year of publication, journal, title, objective and results of the study. March 2013.

From analysing the texts, it can be seen that the year of publication with the highest number of articles was 2007, with 3 publications, followed by 2009, with 2. In 2011, 2006, 2004 and 2000, there was only one publication in each year. However, there were no articles published in the other years.

Among the journals that published the most, the Revista da Escola de Enfermagem da USP stood out, with 4 publications, and the Revista Enfermagem UERJ with 2. Next came the Revista Brasileira de Enfermagem, Revista Ciência, Cuidado e Saúde and Revista de Pesquisa: Cuidado é Fundamental Online, each with 1 publication.

With regard to the objectives proposed by these studies, despite the diversity between them, it was found that most of them aimed to discuss home visits as a health tool; to analyse, discuss and characterise the nurses' work process in the Family Health

Programme, identifying the object, purpose, means and instruments; to understand the characteristics of these nurses' work and the relationship between the processes of empowerment and attrition that are expressed in them; to describe the profile of nurses working in the Family Health Strategy in six municipalities in the southern region of Rio Grande do Sul; to identify the challenges experienced by supervisors in the process of supervising Family Health Teams and to discuss the possibilities of new working practices that contribute to the implementation of the model centred on prevention and health promotion. No articles were identified with the aim of finding out about nurses' work with women in FHS units; only one aimed to find out about the practice of working with families by nurses who work in the Family Health Programme.

The analysis of the articles showed that the nursing work process in the ESF units is of essential importance, since nurses work in health care, in the organisation and management of the unit, reorienting and solidifying practices in this area of care (SILVA; MARTINS, 2009).

According to Schimith and Lima (2009), the nurse's work is more focused on the unit and procedures, carrying out primarily managerial, administrative and collective educational activities, coordinating and supervising activities carried out by community health workers, acting on the basis of the demand that arrives at the units and what the community health workers identify.

Nursing work is almost always the result of the tension between the social and health reality found in the territories and the imposition of targets that fail to address the problems brought by the population (SANTOS; SOARES; CAMPOS, 2007). The organisation of work presents workers with the challenge of meeting targets, taking part in meetings and, at the same time, dealing with unforeseen events, ranging from demands for answers to problems that go beyond the programmes planned for users, to administrative demands that often go beyond the duties previously stipulated for workers. In this sense, in situations of work overload, stress, impotence and physical exhaustion, professional performance is compromised (SILVA; MARTINS, 2009).

Nurses take the individual body as the object of their work, with the aim of intervening in the wear and tear profiles of social groups, and operate in this work process with traditional public health tools, such as the Nursing Consultation and the Home Visit (ERMEL; FRACOLLI, 2006).

In a study on home visits and nursing, it was pointed out that home visits are currently an essential tool for the practice of actions at the primary health care level, especially in the Family Health Strategy. The nurses interviewed in this study perceive home visits as a way of creating conditions that lead to a special closeness with families and the possibility of comprehensive care for the user/family (SANTOS; MORAIS, 2011).

CHAPTER 3

METHODOLOGICAL PATH

3.1 Type of study

To carry out this research, we opted for a descriptive study with a qualitative approach, since, according to Minayo (2010), this approach enables a more in-depth analysis of the object of study, and is concerned with reality, meanings, motives, beliefs, as well as values and attitudes. It is considered the most appropriate to be applied to historical studies, relationships, representations, perceptions, opinions and products of interpretations that subjects make about how they live. This type of approach is ideal for investigating delimited groups, social histories from the perspective of the subjects themselves, "for analysing discourses and documents" (MINAYO, 2010, p. 57).

According to Gil (2010), descriptive research aims to describe the characteristics of a particular population or phenomenon, and is interested in discovering and observing phenomena, seeking to describe and interpret them in order to understand their nature, their composition, as well as the processes that constitute them or those that take place.

In this way, we believe that this method proved to be appropriate for identifying and getting to know the work of nurses and the relationships that are established in the workplace between nurses and the women who work in the ESF units.

3.2 Study Scenario

The study was carried out in the municipality of Santa Maria, located in the central region of the state of Rio Grande do Sul, with an estimated population of 269,740. Of this total, the female population is 138,779, of which 84,327 are of childbearing age, i.e. between 10 and 49 years old, and 63,172 are women between 20 and 59 years old (DATASUS, 2012).

The health system is made up of 32 health units, of which 18 are traditional Basic Health Units (UBS) and 14 are ESF units, with two ESF units having double teams, making a total of 16 teams. The hospital network has 8 hospitals: Hospital de Caridade Astrogildo de Azevedo (HCAA), Hospital Municipal Casa de Saúde, Hospital da Brigada Militar (HBM), Hospital Universitário de Santa Maria (HUSM), Hospital da Guarnição Militar (HGU), Hospital São Francisco, Hospital Dia da UNIMED and Hospital da Base Aérea de Santa Maria (HBASM).

These 16 teams are distributed in the North, South, East, West and Centre regions of the city. The strategy was implemented in 2004, and the places covered by the ESF show better health indices and the population considers the service to be important. Currently, an average of 51,750 people are served, which is only 19.39 per cent of the municipal population (SANTOS, 2011).

In the municipality, there are various programmes offered by the Ministry of Health. The main ones relating to Women's Health are: the National Cervical and Breast Cancer Control Programme, SISCOLO (Cervical Cancer Information System) and SISMAMA (Breast Cancer Information System). These programmes offer pap smears to all women, as well as information on the subject. The municipality also has a reproductive planning assistance programme, which covers everything from raising awareness about family planning to contraceptive methods (condoms, oral and injectable contraceptives, IUDs) and sterilisation, such as tubal ligation and vasectomy. Another important programme in which the municipality participates is the STD and HIV/AIDS Prevention and Control Programme, which raises awareness among professionals and also provides treatment for the syndrome. There is also the SISPRE-NATAL programme, which takes place from the beginning of pregnancy to the consultations after childbirth. The Ministry recommends that a minimum of six antenatal appointments be made, the first of which should take place within the first 120 days of pregnancy. In relation to this programme, which is essential for women's health, the municipality also collects a certain amount of money from its[Q] (COSTA, et al, 2010).

3.3 Study subjects

The research subjects were nurses from the ESF units in the municipality of Santa Maria-RS, who currently make up a group of 16 nurses. Of these, there were a total of 12 nurses who agreed to take part in the research and signed the Informed Consent Form (ICF), belonging to the permanent staff, with one nurse refusing to take part.

They were invited to take part in the research according to their availability, and the dates and times for data collection were scheduled in advance with the participants. The interviews took place in rooms on the premises of the FHS units, at a location chosen by the interviewees.

3.4 Data Collection

Data was collected between May and July 2013, after authorisation from the Research Ethics Committee of the Federal University of Santa Maria (Annex A).

The semi-structured interviews were conducted using a specific script (Appendix A) to facilitate communication between the researcher and the social actors. According to Minayo (2010), the script should serve as a guide for the dialogue, in order to provide flexibility, which contributes to the emergence of other relevant issues. The interview script consisted of two parts: the first sought to characterise the research subjects and the second addressed issues relating to the theme.

The interview was chosen because it provides, as a source of information, data that refers directly to the individual interviewed, which deals with their reflection on reality (subjectivity) and constitutes a representation of reality (MINAYO, 2010).

The interviews were carried out individually, at a place and time scheduled in advance, according to the interviewee's availability. An MP3 audio recorder was used for all the interviews, as a way of guaranteeing greater reliability. However, the recorder was used with the consent of each interviewee. Each interview lasted an average of 30 minutes. In order to maintain the anonymity of the research subjects, they were identified by a code (E.l), determining the interview number.

3.5 Data Analysis

The data was analysed and interpreted using categories, according to Minayo's (2010) proposal for thematic analysis. According to the author, thematic analysis consists of "discovering the nuclei of meaning that make up a communication whose presence means something to the analysed object" (MINAYO, 2010, p. 316).

Initially, the interviews were read and reread. In order to organise and present the results, categories were structured according to the themes that appeared in the interviewees' statements.

According to Minayo (2010), thematic analysis is broken down into three stages: pre-analysis, exploration of the material, treatment of the results obtained and interpretation. In the pre-analysis stage, we returned to the initial research objectives and organised the material to be analysed. Next, a floating reading of each interview was carried out, through which direct and intense contact was made with the material, impregnating it with its content. Subsequently, the interviews were used to produce recording units (key words or phrases), context units (the delimitation of the context in which the recording unit was understood), cut-outs, the form of categorisation, the coding modality and the more general theoretical concepts that guided the analysis (MINAYO, 2010).

In the material exploration stage, the recording and context units that had the same meaning were grouped together. Thematic categories were thus established.

Finally, in the last stage - the treatment of the results obtained and their interpretation - the categories and subcategories that emerged from the material were analysed in relation to the existing literature on the related topics.

3.6 Ethical aspects

As far as ethical aspects are concerned, the research project was registered with the Projects Office (GAP) of the Health Sciences Centre (CCS) at the Federal University of Santa Maria (UFSM), and in the Teaching Information System (SIE), under registration number 033865. It was then submitted to the Centre for Permanent Education of the Santa Maria Health Department (NEPS/SMS), registered on the Brazil Platform and assessed by the Research Ethics Committee (CEP) of the Federal University of Santa Maria (UFSM). It was approved on 20 April 2013, under opinion no. 250.564, under CAAE. 14651313.9.0000.5346, complying with all the ethical precepts defined by Resolution 466/2012 of the National Health Council/MS, on Guidelines and Regulatory Norms for Research Involving Human Beings (BRASIL, 2012b).

In order to comply with the provisions of the aforementioned resolution, the participants in the research were presented with the Free and Informed Consent Form (Appendix B) and, once they had agreed to the form, they signed all the pages, with one copy of the document remaining with the interviewees and the other with the researcher, ensuring their anonymity and supporting their freedom not to take part in the research.

They were also guaranteed the possibility of withdrawing from the study at any time and access to the information they had obtained and the results of the study. In principle, the research did not present any risks or benefits

However, with the subjects' accounts of their subjective relationship with work, there could be an indirect risk of some conflicts and emotional discomfort. If the interview really mobilised this discomfort, it would be terminated, as previously agreed with the researcher, and, if necessary, the interviewee would be referred to a professional from the service.

In order to preserve the identity of those taking part in the research, identification codes were used. As the interviews were recorded, it should be noted that the recordings will be kept by the research supervisor for a period of five years and then destroyed. The researchers undertook to keep the identity of the participants confidential in accordance with the Confidentiality, Privacy and Data Security Agreement (Appendix C), as well as to use the study data for research purposes only.

CHAPTER 4
RESULTS AND DISCUSSION

4.1 Profile of the workers interviewed

Of the 12 nurses interviewed who work in the ESF units in the municipality of Santa Maria, 83.3 per cent were female and 16.6 per cent male, a group predominantly made up of women; 66.6 per cent were aged between 28 and 31; 33.3 per cent were aged between 32 and 36.

The majority of these nurses, 58.3% (7 people), graduated from public universities in Rio Grande do Sul, and the rest from other educational institutions. In terms of time since graduation, the majority (9 nurses) have between 4 and 7 years, 1 has 12 years, 1 has 10 years and another has 8 years. Of these nurses, only 1 has another degree, in Education, and all have *Lato Sensu* training, in one or more specialisation courses, since five listed up to two courses. In the description and distribution of these courses by nursing professional, we found that 33.3 per cent (4) were trained in Family Health and the same percentage in Collective Health; 25 per cent (3) in the Integrated Multiprofessional Residency in the Public Health System (Area of Concentration: Primary Care/Family Health Strategy); 25%, in Intensive Care; 16.6% (2) have specialised in Public Health, 8.3% (1), in Educational Management, and this same percentage, specialised in: Health Education, Technologies Applied to Education, Environmental Education; Urgency, Emergency and Trauma; Integrated Multiprofessional Residency in Hospital Management and Care in the Public Health System (Concentration Area: Chronic Degenerative).

The length of time nurses had worked in nursing prevailed between 1 and 5 years for 58.3% (7) of the nurses; between 6 and 10 years for 33.3% (4) and between 11 and 15 years for 8.3% (1) of the nurses. With regard to the length of time they had been working in the FHS unit, 9 nurses reported having been working for between 1 and 5 years, 2 for between 6 and 10 years and only 1 for between 11 and 15 years.

The statements were analysed according to Minayo's (2010) guidelines, and the following thematic categories emerged: nurses' work with women in the Family Health Strategy; technologies used by nurses at work; the organisation of work with women; difficulties and facilities experienced by nurses when working with women, and nurses' suggestions for improving work with women in the Family Health Strategy.

4.2 Nurses' work with women in Family Health

This category considered the work done by nurses in ESF units within the work process, delimiting it to educational, care and political competences.

4.2.1 Educational practices

Taking into account the various responsibilities of nurses in the FHS unit, we highlight health education, which, although it is the responsibility of all the professionals in the FHS unit, is an activity largely carried out by nurses.

In their study, Leonello and Oliveira (2008) summarised a series of fundamental competences for nurses' educational activities, due to the constant presence of this practice in their care work. These are: promoting comprehensive health care; articulating theory and practice; welcoming and building bonds with the people they assist; recognising themselves and acting as agents for transforming the health reality; recognising and respecting people's autonomy in relation to their lives; respecting common sense knowledge, recognising the incompleteness of professional knowledge; using dialogue as a strategy for transforming the health reality; operating pedagogical techniques that enable dialogue with people; providing people with adequate information; and valuing and exercising intersectoriality in health care.

The competence for educational action of respecting common sense knowledge, recognising the incompleteness of professional knowledge, is a difficult skill to apply in some situations. One of the interviewees explains this difficulty:

"Because they have a different culture. They're not much into medication. Women are more into teas. Homemade things. So the culture is different. Guidance has to be very careful. And I think we have to work on this as professionals, because if we don't, we often end up saying: you take this, this, this and then in her house, she can't eat this, she can't do that and we often generalise. So, as a professional, you also have to look at yourself a little bit, see yourself a little bit so you don't lose sight of that" (E.2).

The hierarchy between scientific and common sense knowledge co-operates with the omnipotence of some health professionals, distancing them from the population they assist. Leonello and Oliveira (2008) state that recognising and respecting common sense knowledge implies recognising the incompleteness of professional knowledge, which does not mean renouncing the scientific knowledge produced. Rather, it means recognising that there are various types of knowledge, including professional knowledge, which is under constant construction and therefore needs to be reformulated, contextualised, confronted and brought closer to other types of knowledge, especially common sense, in order to be transformed into useful knowledge.

One of the ways of practising health education is through the formation of health education groups, in which people with similar characteristics or common needs are interested in sharing and learning knowledge, as well as exchanging ideas about their life experiences.

For Munari et al. (2007), working with groups is directly linked to the dynamics of nursing work, which requires nurses to be directly involved in this type of activity. In addition, these authors point to action centred on the collective as a trend to be followed by various other health actors, to the point of being considered a requirement for those who deal with care.

[1] In order to maintain the originality and integrity of the interviewees' speeches, no textual revision was carried out in terms of agreement or syntax. We have only corrected cases where they do not exist or are not accepted by standard usage. Inverted commas are used to emphasise that it is direct speech.

Leonello and Oliveira (2008) defend the use of health education groups by nurses, as they are an important tool for educational work with collective subjects, especially when a pedagogical perspective of dialogue and participation is adopted.

In the interviewees' speeches, it can be seen that the activities carried out in the groups are geared towards socialising the participants and providing guidance. It was also noted that in these groups it is possible to provide not only education, but also social interaction between the population and the health team.

> *"We hold groups with the women. Social groups so they can talk to each other, they can have a dialogue. [...] Even for them to socialise in some way, many bring a snack, something like that... " (E.2).*

> *"In the group we have with the women, we sometimes do orientation activities. [...] We take advantage of this space to provide guidance to these women. Guidance on health promotion, prevention, the importance of having a cervical exam, breast care, all the guidance for women" (E. 7).*

> *"We started working with them in a Health Group, there's no specific theme, we opened it up and then it became a Health Group, there's no distribution of medicines. It's just a group for guidance, conversation, now we're introducing physical activities and it's directly for women" (E. 10).*

Within the set of health promotion activities, there are operative groups, which are recommended in the national plans for organising health care. They are one of the fields in which health education takes place in primary care and are organised according to the health problem, hypertension, diabetes, adolescence, pregnant women and others (VASCONCELOS; GRILLO; SOARES, 2009). According to the testimonies below, we can see how important the groups are for social inclusion, guidance/education and health promotion.

> *"We've just started a group with women. That's the Health Centre with the Nutrition students. So we want this group to be once a month with the Women's Group, and there's the Hypertensive and Diabetic Group that they're also included in" (E.3).*

> *"The Spine Group is together with the Hypertensive and Diabetic Group, they do their activities and then there's the Hypertensive and Diabetic Group and then there's the Crafts Group as well" (E.8).*

> *"We've tried to reach these women on other occasions. For example, in the hypertension group, we try to raise women's health issues. We have a Childcare Group, [...] then, as the mums were going, we started taking advantage of the weighing day to talk about health issues. The last group was on respiratory infections and the next Childcare Group is going to be on Family Planning, because we see the difficulties they have when we do the pre-consultation. There's also a walking group that the residents run. [...] It's a space to capture this information" (E.12).*

> *"On Fridays, it's prenatal care and the Pregnancy Group. We use the same afternoon to hold the group with the pregnant women who are going to attend the appointments. The Pregnancy Group takes place before the appointments" (E.5).*

"The Health Group covers all age groups, it talks about all subjects" (E.10).

From these statements, it is possible to see significant aspects of the influence of the hegemonic biomedical model in health care, since the names of the Groups refer to the names of diseases and parts of the body. The biomedical model is focused on diseases and specialises in curing the parts of the body that have some pathology, not referring to a biological whole.

In view of this, it is considered that it will only be possible to change this care model if there is a change in the object of care and a reorganisation of health care practice, taking into account the principles of basic care and the SUS: universality, equity, integrality, decentralisation and single command, resolutiveness, regionalisation and hierarchisation, and popular participation (BRASIL, 1990).

Comprehensiveness encompasses health promotion, protection and recovery actions, and groups in FHS units are considered a possibility for health promotion. According to Miranda (2011), the group process can bring participants closer together, provide an informal place to exchange experiences, demonstrate knowledge and facilitate the humanisation of nursing care.

> *"You see them in the social group, building, you know? One talking, for example, about her problem and the other's problem is similar, then they start exchanging. I think this is very motivating for the work. And that's what these actions make possible" (E.2).*
>
> *"We give all the guidance to pregnant women during prenatal care. But when it's a group, we can understand them better, I think there's also a better reception of their needs, each one has a different need, they also help each other, so to speak" (E. 7).*

All the nurses interviewed stressed the importance of holding groups with the community, prioritising their demands, i.e. the doubts and curiosities brought up, and not for some reward offered at the meetings. The speeches show:

> *"It's more a question of them motivating themselves to take part in the groups, without being conditioned. I think people already have articles about this, let's say that people learn on condition, they go to things on condition, that relationship of exchange. I don't think things can be like that, you have to go and learn or want to know about your prenatal care, you know? Because you want to know. Not, 'I'm going there because there's a snack, or because there's a gift at the end, there's a nappy they're going to give me'. Then it's complicated, you don't know if the person is really there. They're absorbing what we're going through [...], it's very complicated" (E.8).*
>
> *"But I assume that you really have to respect that, within that person's reality [...].*

But within what they bring to you, because there's no point in thinking that just the Group, just health education will help, no, maybe not. Maybe they just want a consultation, maybe they just want to be listened to" (E.ll).

The study by Horta et. al. (2009) showed that users' participation in the Groups prevails when they receive some benefit offered at the meetings, such as renewing prescriptions, taking blood pressure, measuring glycaemia and scheduling appointments.

The nurses report that they use the groups as a space for welcoming, bonding and raising awareness of income generation, as they recognise that the lack of employment and income has a direct impact on people's health. It should be remembered that Law No. 8.080 of 19 September 1990, which regulates health actions and services throughout the national territory offered by the SUS, establishes that health is a fundamental right of every human being and, in its third article, places food, housing, basic sanitation, the environment, work, income, education, transport, leisure, access to essential goods and services, among others, as factors that condition health (BRASIL, 1990).

"For income generation, we have the Marias Bonitas Group here, which does all this biscuit work, which they are interested in to generate income, because most of them are heads of household" (E.4).

"We started a group that was demanded by the health workers, a socialising group more geared towards women, it's not closed to women, but we see that the demand, the demand that comes, the people who

participate are women and now some children [...] It's being organised, because it started out as a small business and had a downturn, now we're thinking of restructuring it, thinking of using it as a form of income for the women, but it's starting, slowly... " (E.6).

"We have a *Women's Group, it's a Health Group that discusses, talks about health, beauty. [...] a Women's Group, with an emphasis on health, food health, health... In short, we bring in people to talk about legal issues [...]" (E.5).*

In this way, it is clear to see how much the Groups have a political and economic insertion, not only in the matter of prevention/health promotion, but also in the need to have the Groups as a form of leisure.

4.2. 2Care practices

The nurse is an important member of the care activities in the ESF units, which are carried out by a multi-professional team. According to the Ministry of Health (BRASIL, 2011b), these professionals are trained to provide comprehensive care for women, including prevention, promotion and rehabilitation, as well as guaranteeing the right to health for all women, in all their life cycles. As a professional in the ESF units, nurses need to know a bit about everything, because if they work within the context of their population, they have the most diverse demands, in other words, they cater for different age groups depending on their health needs. The interviewees said that:

> *"In the Strategy, you end up catching the woman at various stages. The phase when she's planning to have children, [...] then she's pregnant and then she's a mum, with this child to accompany her until she's two" (E.ll).*

> *"I do nursing consultations, often based on guidance, on the more preventive side, on guiding women who are hypertensive, women who are diabetic, often women who have family problems [...]. So I do nursing consultations" (E.2).*

In order to carry out women's health care practices, the service is organised through agendas and/or spontaneous demand. The actions carried out by the nurse that stood out were prenatal care, breast and cervical cancer prevention and nursing consultations. Family planning, home visits and

requests for tests, guidance on sexuality and sexually transmitted diseases were also listed.

> *"So, we do the preventive collection, we also do the prenatal consultation [...] we order mammograms, complementary tests, such as: T4, FSH, LH, some others: full blood count. So, we do a bit of everything in the nursing consultation focused on Women's Health" (E.l).*

> *"And it's the nurse who does it: direct prenatal care is done by the nurse, nursing consultations, family planning, collecting cytopathological tests, it's all done by the nurse" (E.4).*

Research into the role of nurses in caring for women in family health centres in the municipality of Diamantino (Mato Grosso do Sul) shows similar data, i.e. cervical cancer prevention prevails, followed by low-risk prenatal care and health education with women as the activities most carried out by nurses in relation to women's health (SEVERINO; COSTA, 2010).

It can be seen that the nurses act as recommended by the Ministry of Health (BRASIL, 2006c) in the control of cervical and breast cancers, prioritising: providing comprehensive care to women; carrying out nursing consultations, collecting preventive examinations and clinical breast examinations; requesting mammography tests and carrying out home care when necessary.

It is the responsibility of the professionals in the ESF unit to provide quality, humanised prenatal and puerperal care. The actions that can be carried out by nurses include: carrying out prenatal consultations for low-risk pregnancies; requesting routine tests; carrying out home visits, when appropriate; carrying out cytopathological tests (BRASIL, 2006b).

We realised that in order to act in accordance with their principles, nurses need to manage their activities, i.e. they need the knowledge and supplies necessary for their work to run smoothly. Therefore, the lack of material is often solved with their commitment.

> *"We ask for material, we say it's missing, we go after it. I finish something, I call the warehouse, there is something. I wait for the lorry to come, I go and get it, you know? We try to make it right" (E. 12).*

Over the years of working in the ESF units, nurses have been shaping and reforming the way nursing is done in public health, both in terms of caring for and promoting people's health.

Planning, organising, executing and evaluating actions, nursing consultations, physical examinations, nursing diagnoses and prescriptions are all tasks that nurses have been responsible for in ESF units. These units demand a closer relationship between the professional and the population and their day-to-day lives, requiring specific skills that were often not required in previous experience (ARAÚJO, 2005).

In the speech transcribed below, it can be seen that nurses predominantly use soft technologies (guidance, conversation) and hard technology material resources (weight checks, pressure checks) for the health production process.

> *"That's specifically it, family planning guidelines; women's health, when women come for the preventive, they're already sought out, we weigh them, check their blood pressure, screen them for these other things, talk to them about their health. The very question of whether they've come for the preventive and are taking the wrong pill, for example, or are without a contraceptive method, the question of guidance on STDs [...]. Handing out contraceptives, for example, is one of the opportunities to*

give advice. Because if we wait for them to come, to the group, something like that, no... We haven't managed to get them to adhere to it yet" (E.12).

According to Merhy (2002), hard technology refers to complex instruments as a whole, encompassing all the equipment for treatments, exams and the organisation of information, and soft technology is produced in live work in action, in a process of interaction and subjectivation relationships, in other words, in the encounter between health worker and user, which makes it possible to produce acceptance, accountability and bonding. It should be emphasised that all technologies are necessary depending on the situation, but at all levels of care, soft technologies need to be present.

Nursing has care as its core competence and responsibility and has the power to move across different fields of knowledge in order to provide this care, or rather, nursing can more intensively establish channels of dialogue with agents from other disciplines and, together, seek out the technologies necessary for care, establishing relationships with the team and the family, acting in the process of transforming reality (MATUMOTO; MISHIMA; PINTO, 2001).

It was noted that nurses are important in ESF units because, as well as attending to users' complaints, their role is also to provide guidance on the health needs of the population. In this sense, it was possible to see that the most common actions carried out by nurses relate to the family, i.e. family planning and care for women and children.

4.2.3 Political practices

Political practice is little described in the scientific literature, because nursing professionals often do not perceive it as permeating other work processes, and even declare themselves to be apolitical. They don't take into account that participating politically doesn't necessarily mean joining a class body, civil rights organisations or a political party. Every moral judgement and attitude that goes with it is a form of political participation, without which it is not possible to be in the world of society (SANNA, 2007).

The entire multi-professional team that works in the ESF unit can be involved in political practice, but nurses stand out because they are the ones who take on the role of leader within the health team, organise and plan the unit's actions and have technical and scientific knowledge on the subject.

The organisation and planning of activities in FHS units involves the participation of the community and professionals in health policy decisions. According to Ordinance 648/2006, two of the characteristics of the work process of the ESF unit team are popular participation in the unit's territories and the strengthening of social control by the health team over the population in the area covered by the programme (BRASIL, 2006a).

Social Control is one of the fundamental principles of the SUS and can be considered an important strategy to guarantee the decentralisation and municipalisation of health; it ensures that the population participates in the process of formulating and controlling health policies (BRASIL, 1990). It can be defined as the "[...] capacity that civil society has to interfere in public management, guiding the actions of the state and state spending towards the interests of the community [...]" (CORREIA, 2000, p.53).

In order to exercise social control over the SUS, the Health Councils and Conferences were created as vital spaces in the three spheres of government: national, state and municipal. They work to draw up strategies and control the implementation of health policy. Health Conferences are held at least every four years, through a National Conference and various State and Municipal Conferences, providing opportunities to discuss and analyse the general health situation of the population and establishing guidelines for the operation of SUS health services.

Health Councils, on the other hand, are defined as deliberative and permanent collegiate bodies made up of government representatives, service providers, health professionals and users, with users being represented on an equal basis with other segments (BRASIL, 1990b). In addition to the Municipal Councils, there is another option, the Local Councils, which are hierarchically prior to the Municipal Health Councils and are made up of representatives from neighbourhoods and health professionals, especially in places where there are FHS units.

Of the nurses interviewed in this study, only one mentioned his political activity:

> *"We take part in the Local Health Council, there's a health worker who is a member, and I'm an alternate member of the Local Council. And we always try to involve the management in everything we can. We call the other units when necessary. We call them if there's anything wrong [...] We try to establish partnerships here and especially with the other services. And we've tried to enlighten the community" (E. 12).*

According to Arantes et al. (2007), nurses can contribute directly to the search for effective social control, while carrying out their managerial, educational and basic care functions.

> We believe that nurses can play an important role in building and strengthening social control, especially those who work in primary health care units, as they are in direct contact with the population that uses the services and, to a large extent, have a role in articulating both the activities carried out and the different workers involved in the process of producing health actions (ARANTES et al., 2007, p. 471).

In this way, nurses in ESF units have a relevant duty towards the population they serve, but not only in terms of health needs, but also to involve the population in the search for their health needs, making them citizens who are committed to self-care and the care of others. However, it encourages government officials to seek to fulfil the real needs of the population.

4.3 Technologies used by nurses at work

Merhy (2007) defines technology as a set of knowledge and actions applied to the production of something, also including the knowledge used in the production of unique products in health services, as well as the knowledge that operates to organise human and inter-human actions in production processes. This knowledge can be materialised in machines and instruments - hard technologies; structured knowledge and practices - soft-hard technologies - and living work/production of services/approach to care (ways of producing acceptance, bonding and accountability) - soft technologies (FRANCO; MERHY, 2007). According to Gomes (2011), the health practices of the professionals in the ESF unit must combine technologies capable of guiding the care of individuals and families, from newborns to the elderly, whether healthy or sick, prioritising the production of care.

The use of relationship technologies, classified as soft technologies, in health work involves the processes of welcoming, bonding and comprehensive care as managers of health actions. The nurse is the professional who has the space to provide care, receive and assist the user, and soft technologies are essential to the progress of the work process.

Reception is a way of universalising user access to the Family Health Unit (USF) and the health system network, i.e. opening the unit's doors to all clients who need them. The link, in turn, is based on establishing a reference for users to a given health team of workers and making them responsible for providing care (FRANCO; MERHY, 2007).

The nurses interviewed referred to welcoming only in terms of its organisational logic, i.e. a system for scheduling appointments, which allows for the organisation of scheduled demand and meeting free daily demand. In this sense, welcoming appears in ESF units, according to certain statements:

> *"We have the appointments, by free demand that they seek care in the unit, like the reception, and we also have the bookings. There are appointments for preventive examinations, cervical examinations, which we do once a week [...]" (E. 7).*

> *"We have the normal appointments for women's care, we take a form or we welcome them" (E.9).*

According to the Ministry of Health, welcoming is:

> The reception of the user, from the moment they arrive, taking full responsibility for them, listening to their complaints, allowing them to express their concerns, anxieties and, at the same time, setting the necessary limits, guaranteeing resolutive care and liaising with other health services for continuity of care when necessary (BRASIL, 2004, p. 43).

As a result, it was found that an access system is applied to the ESF units, which implements the idea of booking scheduled appointments associated with welcoming free demand. This mechanism involves improving the service provided and reducing the difficulties users have in accessing the units, in other words, it guarantees accessibility, but not the reception recommended by the Ministry of Health.

This emphasises the importance of welcoming any and all users who come to the unit looking for help, as well as the ability of the Basic Health Unit to meet a large part of people's health problems and needs, acting as an articulator between the various technologies available for basic care (BRASIL, 201 Id).

In the study by Leonello and Oliveira (2008), the interviewees saw welcoming as a way of recognising and knowing how to listen to people's health needs. It is therefore known that the exercise of listening, through welcoming, requires that the health professional likewise become involved and committed to the subjects and their needs. This involvement and commitment can be demonstrated by the bond.

Building bonds means maintaining close and clear relationships with the people being cared for, being sensitive to their suffering, facilitating the construction of their autonomy, taking responsibility for their care and knowing how to relate to and integrate with these people, in the health service itself and in the community (MERHY, 1994). This notion can also be seen in the interviewees' statements:

> *"So I've been trying to work on looking at the person, looking at the woman and really seeing what she's looking for in that service, because often it's not just what we're offering that she's looking for" (E.2).*

> *"And through conversation, a qualified consultation, a well-crafted welcome. I try to listen beyond what they bring, sometimes they say: 'I just want to do the injection', no more, what else, how's your life? Your children, your husband? Don't you have any? How's life? Your work? Then they leave here happy and in a little while they're coming back, looking for you. I've noticed this with many people. Now, if you don't, if you just hand them the pill, more or less, without looking at their face, in a while that person won't come back to you, you'll lose them, they'll go to another unit where they can be seen. So, little by little, we're changing, I think it takes time, I've been here for a year and a half, it's still a short time, but I think there have already been some gains" (E.6).*

> *"And the question of being able to do other activities that involve the whole unit; the month of the June festival, we do the June festival for the community; carnival, we try to do a party that reminds them of it. So, I mean, it's also a way for them to get to know the unit, to come here at other times, not just when they need to be treated or cured. But also to come for other entertainment. Now, next week, there's the Solidarity event, about the Warm Clothing Campaign we ran, with everything we collected. We're going to open the unit in one shift just to do the Solidarity clothesline. So, I mean, it's a way for you to bring families in need together, for them to realise that the Unit isn't just for treating illness, but that it's also for creating this bond with them" (E.ll).*

The nurse uses strategies to create a bond with the community, such as listening to complaints, seeking to get closer to the user in a way that generates a positive relationship with the community.

trust, respect and empathy, so that they participate. It also organises the service with activities that involve all the professionals in the unit and the users, so that they become familiar with the services provided. Forming a bond leads to a closer relationship between the team and the community, which favours adherence to health services.

Interviewee E. 11's speech shows the nurse's concern to demonstrate to users that they shouldn't go to the unit just to cure/treat the disease, but rather to prevent it. They are thus trying to show that the object of their work is not the disease, but rather the risk factors and specific aggravations of the disease and its modes of transmission. The search for detachment from the biomedical model, which still intervenes in health care, is clear.

Access, welcoming and bonding, as technological resources, represent a relationship established between workers and users, so that health actions are more welcoming, agile and resolutive (COELHO; JORGE, 2009).

In ESF units, nurses carry out various types of actions in their caring dimension for women, from pregnancy to old age, providing not only access, but also consolidating bonds, welcoming, and contributing to problem-solving, disease prevention and health promotion.

The bond, as a light technology of relationships in the ESF, is based on the principle that health workers should establish responsibility for the area they are assigned to; consequently, there is an interaction that generates bonds, 'ties', between health workers and users, which is necessary for the technological mechanism for carrying out the work, in accordance with the guidelines that guide the practice of the ESF (BRASIL, 1997).

These testimonies show that the bond is fundamental to ensuring bonds of complicity, affinity and trust, mediating the relationship between professional and user:

> *"The bond we have makes it easier, because you get to know them. Because the ESF is a defined area, so generally, from one year to the next, it's always going to be the same people. Most of them will be the same, so you already create that bond for us to do our work" (E.4).*
>
> *"A consultation is done along with the collection, it's not done, I just go there and collect it and it's done. And it's a consultation that takes time, some take up to an hour, forty minutes... Some are a bit quicker, it depends on the woman's situation and their availability and the bond that is forming. I realise that this is starting to happen, because they had a great bond with the other nurses who had been there longer. And now they're getting to know me [...]" (E. 6).*

The formation of bonds in ESF units is evident when E.4 points out that the professionals already know the population located in the area defined for their work, and identify the people and families to which they belong. In this way, they establish a partnership of trust, commitment and empathy with the population, favouring the referral of their health problems so that they can be solved.

Nurses in the ESF units use the nursing consultation to facilitate monitoring women's health and forming a bond. Nursing consultations are the exclusive responsibility of nurses. The Law on Professional Practice - No. 7,498 of 25 June 1986 - legitimises nurses to fully exercise their activity with individuals, families and the community, in hospital, outpatient and home settings or in private practice (BRASIL, 1986).

Interviewee E.6 says that the nursing consultation in Women's Health allows for the creation of a bond between nurse and user. At this point, the professional seeks to get closer to the woman, not worrying about the length of the consultation, but rather promoting a dialogue so that she can expose her anxieties, experiences and doubts.

4.4 Organising work with women

The organisation of services in ESF units and the planning of activities are part of the nurse's duties. Therefore, in order to carry out some activities, the organisation is done by means of agendas establishing days and/or periods in order to provide care to women (preventive collection, nursing and prenatal consultations with guidance on family planning, sexually transmitted diseases (STDs), sexuality). When they're not attending by appointment, they follow free demand.

> *"We have the appointment for the cytopathological test, which is then collected, breast exams and guidance on sexuality, family planning, which is then provided by the nurses. [...] There's prenatal care, where if there's a Beta, we call, we collect, we ask for the first tests and we schedule all the subsequent appointments, which are interspersed between the doctor and the nurse" (E.9).*

In nurses' day-to-day work, there is a search for appropriate planning for the organisation of their work, with the aim of providing users with effective and efficient care.

The work of caring for women is carried out by a multi-professional team. The interviewees were unanimous in saying that all the professionals in the team are involved in providing care for women. Some units have the minimum team: doctor, nurse, nursing assistant and community health workers, while others have an expanded team, including a dentist and oral health worker. The important participation of residents and academics from various areas of health (nutrition, occupational therapy, social workers, physiotherapy and nursing) was also mentioned as support for the service.

> *"And the nurse, then there's the resident nurse, I have the nursing technician. The nurse does the nursing consultations, the appointments, you name it. The nursing technician does the procedures related to these consultations, consultations with the doctor, the doctor also gets involved; the health agents, in the active search for some woman, because she didn't come for the cytopathological test (CP), there was some alteration in the cytopathological test (CP). I also have a resident nutritionist and a social worker [...] They have an appointment with the nutritionist. In the groups, the nutritionist advises on healthy eating, the social worker on the legal side, on some problem of violence, something like that. So that's what's done" (E.5).*

> *"I think the whole team is involved in caring for women, the doctor, the nurse, the technician and the community health workers too [...]. When we need to carry out an active search, we have a lot of accessibility with them in this respect. I believe that all the professionals are involved [...]" (E. 7).*

> *"Our team is very good. So much so that it's not everywhere that the doctor and nurse do joint prenatal care. They do ours, we do it together, and the dentist does dental prenatal care. All our pregnant women go through*
>
> *dentist. [...] The basic team, which is a doctor, nurse and dentist, everyone provides this care for women, which is a little different when you're pregnant" (E.9).*

The relevance of teamwork in the ESF unit is due to the aspect of comprehensive care for individuals and families; its purpose is to obtain results on the different factors that interfere in the health-disease process of individuals and families in a territory. Comprehensiveness is one of the doctrinal principles of the SUS and is an important strategy for implementing the new model proposed in the SUS (ARAÚJO; ROCHA, 2007).

In this way, the comprehensive approach to individuals and families is produced by the sum of the different perspectives of the health workers who make up the ESF unit. In this way, a greater impact can be achieved on the different determinants and conditioning factors that affect the health-disease process (FRANCO; MERHY, 2007).

The statements made by interviewees E.7 and E.9 show that teamwork takes place in the sense of the division of responsibilities between its members, in which everyone participates with their specialities, cooperating for the quality of the actions provided in the search for comprehensive health care. According to the Ministry of Health, teamwork is one of the most important characteristics of the ESF, as it is one of the most important presuppositions for reorganising the work process and as a possibility for a more comprehensive and resolutive approach (BRASIL, 2001b). The professionals in the team are called upon to carry out their profession in a collective work process, the product of which must be the result of work that is forged with the specific contribution of the various professional areas or areas of knowledge. The aim is for team members to be able to "get to know and analyse their work, checking their specific duties and those of the group, in the unit, at home and in the community, as well as sharing knowledge and information" (BRASIL, 2001c, p.74).

In the speeches of the interviewees, there are references to work situations that highlight the articulation of actions and the delimitation of professional roles. In a way, they show that at certain moments in their work

work, they seek out other members of the team to exchange information, mainly with a view to clarifying doubts.

> *"Firstly, as I said, the health agents... "Firstly, as I said, the health agents, they go to the houses, they have access to go into the houses, see the woman, the daughter, the granddaughter, they have this access to people; me, as a nurse, in those cases I mentioned: Women's Groups, prenatal care, preventive care, breast exams; that part, the doctor and I do the same thing: we do medical consultations, prenatal care, preventive care, I do it. But we give referrals to specialists if necessary. A mastologist, a gynaecologist or some other test he'll have to order, so he's involved in that part; and the nursing technician we have, who's involved directly and indirectly, he sees the signs, a woman comes to see him, he asks about the preventive test and refers her to us for an appointment, he's involved in this way of making appointments, the signs to look out for when your blood pressure is high, you're not taking care of yourself, then we all... When he looks and sees an altered HGT, he already says: "Wow, this one is... Let's see with Nutrition, let's see with the nurse, let's see with the doctor what we can do"' (E.3).*

> *"The health agent, he does the active search, guidance. The nurse does prenatal care, consults with pregnant women, in short... nursing consultations. The doctor also provides prenatal care when necessary. The dentist does the assessments. And when we have Women's Groups, we close the door and everyone goes. So everyone is always involved, always working together, at least that's our aim here, not to segment the work, where there's... Not least because it's everyone's job to work*

collectively in the ESF. So we try, if there's a group, if there's counselling at a school, we close up and everyone goes, because there's always going to be someone who has a different or new counselling to give. The dentist is one, the agent is another, the doctor is another, the technician is another, so everyone gets involved" (E.10).

"The whole team, I think, regardless of any profession. There's nutrition, there are physiotherapy students, each user has their own peculiarities, so we end up using the professionals we have. But it's nice for us to be able to exchange with them and for each of them to be able to do their different activities. Of course, nursing ends up using a bit more of the devices, a bit more than dentistry, for example. But anyway, it's because it's part of the profession, part of the centre. So everyone does it. Women end up going through all the professionals here" (E.ll).

It can thus be seen that the interaction between professionals and the unity of their work is part of teamwork. They endeavour to carry out their work collectively; although there is a division of duties between the professionals, there is a sharing of actions.

4.5 Difficulties and facilities experienced by nurses when working with women

During this study, several situations of difficulty experienced by nurses with regard to working with women were reported. The following table summarises these situations:

Table 1 - Distribution of situations of difficulty experienced by nurses in FHS units, Santa Maria/RS, 2013

Work Situations Experienced	No. of nurses
Lack of materials and financial resources	3
Difficulty accessing the ESF unit	3
Women's low attendance at preventive examinations	2
Lack of support from management	2
Incompatible unit opening hours for working women	2
Women's participation in groups	2
The types of contraceptives offered to women	2
Nomadic families	2
Attendance in de-territorialised areas without health workers	2
Lack of medication (folic acid)	2
Women missing appointments	1
Work Situations Experienced	No. of nurses
Difficulty for women to understand contraceptive use	1
Women don't seek services	1
Women don't adhere to treatment	1
Delayed referrals to specialities	1
Population vulnerability	1
Inadequate physical structure of the ESF unit	1
Women's dependence on men, violence in the home	1

Among these situations, the interviewees say they face a lack of materials, especially office supplies, problems with the physical structure and financial resources.

"We have difficulties in the physical area. Because we could be doing a lot more [...]. Sometimes, the colleague is downstairs and I'm here, I could be doing a lot more, I say 'better utilised'..." (E.4).

"[...] there's no material, like, for groups, we don't have the resources. Often, if you want to do something prettier, something that calls out, you have to take it out of your own pocket, like balloons, ribbons, some treat to bring or some snack to bring, or you have to ask for it; often, you can't get it. So these are the difficulties of not having the resources. As the Strategy is geared towards prevention and promotion, we should be much more involved in groups, in things, than clinically in the Unit. We often end up not doing this because, good or bad, we need something to get their attention. As well as talking, inviting, you have to make a little card, you have to make an invitation, you have to have the day written down, because they might forget" (E.6).

In relation to inadequate physical structure, the study carried out by Madeira (2009) also addresses problems with physical space in a Family Health Unit, which has a limited physical area for all the activities carried out. This reality is also pointed out by Cunha et al. (2013): in their research, it appears as one of the main impediments that make work difficult, along with the lack of financial resources, procedural materials, shortage of medicines and low pay. Severino and Costa (2010) and Pinto (2008), in their studies, cited the unavailability of materials as difficulties in carrying out day-to-day work activities. Unfortunately, these difficulties are recurrent in ESF units and hinder the quality of the services offered.

Other statements refer to the difficulty women have in accessing the ESF unit.

"One thing I find very difficult is the distance involved. [...] It's very difficult, because then it's a matter of calling the Secretariat to get to where they are. Because it's so far away, I can't get there. [...] I need the car; I have a group with the women, or I have some other activity to do, sometimes the issue of home visits as well. When a woman or a man asks, I don't have a car available, so I often have to call the Secretariat, book it for another day, then people wait, or I often have to wait an hour, half an hour for the car to arrive at the unit" (E.2).

"We have an area, two areas, that are far from the Strategy and that we notice, from there, that the women don't come to the activities very often. [...] Because they depend on the bus, the bus timetables are bad; to come on foot, the roads are bad, there's a lot of mud. So we notice that it's often difficult to get there because they're far away" (E. 6).

"The distance they have to travel is also a difficulty, access is a difficulty, because there aren't buses all the time. There's a bus every six hours, not every six minutes. The unit is relatively far away, because it's not ten blocks, it's not five blocks, it's ten kilometres, it's five kilometres. Sometimes it's two or three kilometres from one house to another, so that's the difficulty" (E.10).

Similarly, this difficulty is pointed out by other studies that deal with the obstacles faced by professionals in carrying out their work in the ESF unit. Madeira (2009) points out that the area's vast geographical territory, isolation and the distance from the localities to the health unit make it difficult for the population to get there, and this difficulty is reinforced by the inflexibility of bus timetables. Lopes and Marcon (2012) report that there are no vehicles for travelling to the homes; the car for the professionals is made available only once a week for each team. Normally, there are a large number of families to be visited, requiring the professionals to carefully select the most urgent cases, often prioritising those with the greatest need for home monitoring. However, this condition may be limited to caring for the person who is suffering and not all the members of the family.

The speeches emphasise that the professionals working in the ESF unit have faced difficulties in providing adequate care to users. The problem of access has affected the travelling of both users to health professionals and health professionals to users. The lack of transport was mentioned by the nurses, as its absence makes it impossible to carry out activities properly, such as home care, which requires its use due to the distance between homes and the unit. Users' difficulties are associated with the geographical difficulty of locating the Unit, which is far from their homes, the precarious bus timetables and the infrastructure of the roads, which make it impossible to access the services.

Two interviewees were demotivated by the lack of management support and professional responsibility.

> *"So, these things make it a bit difficult to work, and when we don't have this support from management. [...] But I mean management as a whole, you know? It doesn't really give us the support we need to move forward with this kind of work, because the logic of the PSF is to work more on prevention and health promotion and not so much on the curative side. But it seems that this curative part is so... No, it seems to be so strong that we can't move forward in the work process [...]. So this makes us a little discouraged a lot of the time, because we try to do it, you want to do it and you don't have the support, we go after it, we know it doesn't just depend on us, because there's the professional issue, the professional has to want to do this kind of activity with the women, but if you don't have support behind you, you can't do it either. So there's the professional thing, and there's a bit of management too" (E.2).*
>
> *"And the working relationship, the management that doesn't prioritise public health today is very complicated" (E.10).*

It can be seen that the difficulty of management support makes nurses feel demotivated about their work, since they see the problems, they want to solve them, they feel like taking more action, but without the SUS managers taking up the issue, they end up feeling discouraged.

Primary Care is a set of health actions, both individual and collective, that covers health promotion, prevention, recovery and rehabilitation of the most common diseases and illnesses. In this way, it moves away from the curative model towards preventative and rehabilitative actions. Interviewee E.2's speech exposes the difficulty nurses face in applying the care model laid down in health policies for primary care, which prioritises health promotion and surveillance.

With regard to family planning in the ESF units, two nurses reported difficulties in offering contraceptives to women.

> *"[...] The contraceptives, we only have the quarterly, the quarterly injectable, the progesterone and the Microvlar contraceptive, and that's it! And the IUD, we send it to her if she wants to have it fitted [...]. What I'm referring to is that we could have, for example, a better contraceptive for teenagers, something better that's on the market, for example, the patch, some different things" (E.4).*
> *"Another difficulty: we don't have a pill for teenagers [...]. What you get today, Microvlar or the three-month injection [...] (E.12).*

Therefore, it can be seen that the services provided are limited in terms of not offering contraceptive methods with different dosages and application techniques. It is known that, in general, adolescents can use most of the contraceptive methods available. However, some methods are more appropriate than others at this stage of life.

When carrying out activities with women in the ESF units, the nurses mentioned some of the facilities they found at work, which are shown in Table 2.

Table 2 - Distribution of facility situations experienced by nurses at FHS units, Santa Maria/RS, 2013.

Work Situations Experienced	No. of nurses who answered
Bonding with patients	4
The presence of the community health worker	4
Gender issue	4
Mature women	2
Service in the unit is well organised	1
0 good team relationships	1
Improvements to the Women's Health room	1

It can be seen that the facilities that predominated were the formation of a bond between the nurse and the users, the presence of the community health agent and the gender issue, according to the speeches transcribed below.

> *"Look, the easiest thing is that they've already learnt, they've already created a bond. So they come in here and say 'I want to talk to you a bit'. The first thing they say is 'I want to talk to you a bit'. Then we do a little nursing consultation and sometimes they just want to ask a question, something, so that's easy" (E.5).*

> *"People trivialise the collection of preventive tests; for me it's the richest consultation a woman has. Especially because if she talks about sex, she talks about how she feels about sex, she can talk about anything else. And so, here, they talk about everything, if they like it, if they don't like it, if they want it, if they don't want it, if they have a lover, if they don't have a lover, and we know the most intimate things about those women. So, when you have that, you get a very good bond with these women" (E.9).*

> *"I think it's easy to create a bond with her. [...] This issue of the bond with the woman, you have more than with the man, who only comes when he needs it. Women come more to the appointment just to talk... So this part of the bond with women is a little easier" (E.11).*

In their study, Lopes and Marcon (2012) also found the bond to be the main facility. They pointed out that a good bond makes it easier to pass on guidance and invest in disease prevention. However, Severino and Costa (2010) identified the lack of a bond with women as a major difficulty for nurses, not least because of the change of nurses, which jeopardises care.

In the nurses' speeches, reference is made to the nursing consultation as an activity that facilitates building a bond. The nursing consultation is a private activity of the nurse, which is part of a series of attributions of the professional who works in the ESF units. It is supported by the current legislation on Professional Nursing Practice (Law 7498/86) and ensured by the Federal Nursing Council (Resolution 358/2009), which provides for the systematisation of nursing care and the implementation of the nursing process in public and private environments where professional nursing care takes place (BRASIL, 1986; BRASIL, 2009c).

The nursing process is a systematised method that nurses use to organise their ideas and information in order to better plan the care provided to their clients. One of the objectives of the nursing consultation, as an important stage in the nurse's work process, is to bring the client closer to and interact with the environment in which they live, with the aim of achieving maximum well-being, offering them opportunities to achieve autonomy and feel self-realised (ZAGONEL, 2001).

In interviewee E.5's speech, the word "consultinha" shows a certain disdain, a failure by the professional to value a specific nursing activity. This shows that nurses sometimes don't take ownership of a practice that is a priority in their professional practice.

The support provided by the CHAs was mentioned by the nurses as crucial to the development of their work:

> *"The facilities I think are the fact that we are a strategy and have some health workers. And having these people to support us, to bring these women, to look for them, because it's a closed area, it was supposed to be in reality... " (E.6).*

> *"Facilities... I think that when we have, for example, a professional community health worker, our service becomes easier, so to speak. Because they often book the preventive examinations and we know that there are those who miss them, so they already do it, they already see who missed that day and they already do the active search for that woman, so they can reschedule and find out why she didn't come to collect it. So it makes your job with the community health agent a lot easier" (E. 7).*

> *"The community agents are from the area, they know a lot of the people, they're neighbours. [...] So they talk, sometimes they're even compadres, they know everyone in the area, they get on well. All the agents get on well with the public in each micro-area. And if they call people, mobilise them, listen to them, see them, they have credibility. So that's how easy it is to work with them" (E.10).*

> *"The work of the agents also helps a lot. So, mainly to actively seek out patients, pregnant women, for example. So-and-so didn't come to her appointment, she goes to see what happened; so that's very important" (E.12).*

Santana et al. (2009), in a study on CHWs, reported that this professional plays a significant role in the work process of the FHS unit, as they act as a link between the community and the other members of the Family Health team, mainly because of the bond they must establish with the family, which can provide trust, solidarity and respect, fundamental characteristics in health promotion. This enables a link to be made between technical and scientific information and popular knowledge, favouring users' access to health services.

The gender issue was highlighted by the nurses as a facilitating aspect in forming a bond and carrying out preventive examinations, because they often seek not just a consultation, but a professional with whom they can feel more at ease, to talk about their difficulties, doubts, problems, etc.

> *"Even on this issue of women's health, they'd rather talk to me than see a doctor. So, often, I'm in the screening area or doing something else, and even when they come to see the doctor, they say: 'Oh, I've got a little problem down there, it's like this, like this...' So, you take the opportunity to go and see me and say it. "So, you take advantage of the fact that you're going to see the doctor and you say: 'Oh, but I'm ashamed'; so, you know, they come, they still come to us. So it's very gratifying" (E.*

1).

"I'm the only one who does the preventive, the doctor doesn't collect it. Except in a few cases, like me being a man, there are many women who are embarrassed. Then we have to use common sense too, to be able to provide this service. So, I often tell the doctor that the woman doesn't want to do the screening with me, and she ends up doing it. So she does it too, but to a lesser extent, because I end up taking on more of this service. But this is very rare, most women accept it calmly, without any problems" (E.2).

"Women talk more, they expose themselves more, they can... So that's one of the things that makes it easier; something that with men you don't make that contact, that conversation, they don't open up, it's not possible. With women, it's easier" (E.9).

"And because we're also women nurses, I think it makes it much easier for you to understand. So even if, several times, we find ourselves at a point where we don't know how to answer all the questions, something like that, but being a woman makes it a little easier" (E.ll).

According to the study carried out by Montenegro (2010), nurses showed that being a woman facilitates their relationship with users, especially when it comes to meeting women's health needs.

It also interferes with the work of primary care, since it is permeated by social relationships that often go beyond technical competence in the performance of their duties.

4.5.1 Strategies used to deal with the difficulties and facilities of the job

This subsection describes the strategies that nurses use to deal with the facilities/difficulties in their work with women in ESF units.

The interviewees pointed to a series of strategies for attending to women's health, such as: active search, group care, follow-up, involvement, partnerships with universities, facilitating access to the service, team meetings, leaving the door open to the service whenever necessary and a waiting room.

In the study by Severino and Costa (2010), the strategies employed by nurses to motivate women to undergo cervical cancer screening were the right to take part in prize draws, beauty parlours and gifts from shops. They say that in this way they encourage the female population to take the test, and this creates a moment of bonding with the women.

Analysing the speeches, it emerged that there is a predominance of the use of search

with the participation of the ACS.

> *"One of the strategies is the facility we have in the case of health agents, who actively seek out women, who talk to them. When it comes to prenatal care, why they're not going. We have a notebook with the frequency. So, every month I check up on them, and then we try to go after those who are absent, and the same thing with Women's Health, the issue of exams, these complementary exams, everything, they talk to me and they see the case and pass it on to me and, if there's anything, we call them" (E.l).*

> *"The strategy I use is the support of the community agents as well. Because the woman has her monthly appointment. So they're the ones who follow up the rest of the month and I'm always in contact with them asking: 'How is that pregnant woman, how is the pregnant woman in your area, did you go there? How is she?'" (E.2).*

> *"What we use as a strategy here are the health agents. [...] The health agents help with preventive care, they help with mammograms, if they're overdue we let them know: 'oh, this lady hasn't had one in three years, go and get it', they go and get it for us. There's the Women's Group, they send out invitations; there's Nutrition, the appointments, they let people know that Nutrition is offering appointments" (E.3).*

> *"Generally, because we have the community health agent, we do the active search. So, if a woman has had a preventive test altered, if she's had something like that, we go after her. That woman who we know is suffering from violence, something like that, we go and visit her [...]" (E.ll).*

In family health units, the nurse adds coordination, guidance and supervision of the CHW's actions to their work process. This professional collaborates with the nurse in women's health care, in the active search for those who miss prenatal examinations and appointments, in home visits, in the monthly monitoring of pregnant women and in passing on information about activities taking place in the unit.

4.6Nurses ' suggestions for improving work with women in the Family Health Strategy

The suggestions made by the nurses revealed their needs in relation to their work, so that they can improve the quality of the service offered to the community. Among the suggestions made by the nurses, those relating to the formation of more women's/health groups stood out, thus making it possible to expand health promotion.

> *"Look, my suggestion would be for them to participate more in the groups. [...] That there should be an attraction, an investment from the municipal administration, so that we can make groups. [...] So, a financial incentive, to buy material, even for us*

to carry out this work" (E.5).

"We could implement more groups, for example, I think, because women often find it difficult to join the group. Suddenly, some active search, some invitation, something that they can come to the unit for" (E. 7).

The nurses suggest greater incentives for holding groups, as they know that these are the main actions carried out with a focus on health promotion. These spaces provide development for all those involved, through the opportunity to interfere creatively in the health-disease process and to enrich their varied knowledge.

Another suggestion made by the nurses was to have more human, material and financial resources. According to them, all these points make it difficult to offer improvements in the service.

"Maybe it's a bit more resources. [...] So the lack of resources, material, equipment. Sometimes we don't have a shirt to put on the patient. So we kind of improvise, try to... Sometimes, on a cold day, we don't have a heater for you to do the examination so that the woman is more relaxed. So it's more a question of a lack of material resources" (E. 1).

"There's no receptionist here, we've already told the Secretariat that, since I've been here, I've wanted a receptionist. [...] If we could get a receptionist, it would help us to do the service, [...] a printer to make folders, everything we print at home or everything that's educational, colourful, is brought by Nutrition. So the part that we would need is more material to work in a different way, but on a day-to-day basis it's more or less fine. What's missing: a reception professional and educational material. I think these things would improve if we had them" (E.3).

"We would need more qualified people, a psychologist, a social worker. [...] A lot of the demands here are more social [...]" (E.6).

"I think the issue that every site has is human resources. [...] But the lack of human resources means that you can't attend to these 15,000 people and reach the majority of the homes you'd like to. So I think the main point is that it's not just here, it's the whole municipality, the whole hospital, I know there is. It's never going to be right. So that's the basic point. Well, to have the ideal number of human resources, of nurses, to attend to this fifteen thousand. Then you can do other activities, you can open up more spaces for visits, you know? " (E.ll).

In their speeches, the interviewees indicated that investments in improvements should be made available in these FHS units, where professionals should provide solutions, comprehensive care and continuity of care for the population. Some suggestions are related to working with and empowering the community. In this sense, communication and the media are relatively important as a strategy for bringing professionals closer to the community.

> *"I think working with the community, you know? Talking to the community, going out. One day we spoke to a chap from the community radio station, and he opened up a space for us. For us to talk, for us to explain, because we see that people don't have information, they lack basic information. And sometimes one person asks another and the other doesn't know and says something rubbish. [...] I think that by enlightening the community, we can even make these demands, to get material, to improve the structure. It's the community that has the strength to ask for this, to influence the management in this direction. So I think that's one of the fundamental things. And this rapprochement with the community and training is basic" (E. 12).*

> *"The question of empowerment, which sometimes we end up with, and I think a lot in the preventive collection appointment, we have this chance, you know? To talk about rights, because sometimes there's a complaint of violence. Sometimes verbal, sometimes even sexual, it comes up a lot in the preventive. You talk to these women about their rights, what services are available that can help. Even we sometimes have someone who is older, who hasn't studied, who can't read, and you encourage them. We have to be involved in family health, we have to try to broaden our perspective [...] Last year, during a conversation with NEMGeP (Centre for Studies on Women, Gender and Public Policies) at UFSM, the girls were here. We managed to hold a meeting with sixty women on a Saturday, with a video... it was really nice. It was really empowering, and many of them come, fight for the community and take part. So that's interesting, it keeps them alive. Sometimes they have another objective, something else... Sometimes it's not possible to talk to the women about the clinical side, that's what the doctor does. The nurse looks at it differently, it has to be different" (E.9).*

Interviewee E.9's statement about empowerment shows that it is an indispensable component in health promotion. Therefore, "empowerment" is not about transferring power, it is about building the capacity to make decisions to improve living conditions and have control over the situation of social exclusion, resulting in a better quality of life. (OLIVEIRA et al. 2011, p. 285).

Thus, the nurses' suggestions are many and are based on their experiences, their difficulties in caring for women and their work process. The nurses know how much power the community has to make demands, but they only use it when they really need it or when an extreme situation occurs. In this way, nurses realise that the community is the main ally in achieving goals and that work can only happen if everyone has the same objective

CHAPTER 5

FINAL CONSIDERATIONS

The path taken in this research provided an opportunity to learn about and analyse the work of nurses with women in the Family Health Strategy Units of Santa Maria/RS, in order to understand their practices and the technologies used to carry out their work. It also made it possible to identify the facilities, difficulties and strategies used by nurses to work with women in these units.

During the data collection, it was possible to see that the interviews sometimes took on the character of nurses letting off steam, as they used the moment to express the feelings that the work brings, sometimes of motivation, due to the return of the users, sometimes of incapacity, discouragement and lack of support for the problems they face.

In the course of analysing the data, it was possible to understand that the nurses are committed to various practices in their work with women - care, educational and political practices, which show the extent of their field of work in Women's Health. The work is organised through a multi-professional team, in which all the professionals get involved, i.e. they try to carry out collective, rather than segmented, work. The team makes use of technological resources, such as welcoming and bonding, to offer a more organised and resolutive service to its users, and groups, to promote health and strengthen the bonds between professional and user, a valuable tactic in ESF units for adherence to services.

In care practice, the main activities carried out were prenatal care, breast and cervical cancer prevention and nursing consultations, all of which provide women with the opportunity to receive guidance, clear up doubts and empower them. Family planning, home visits, test requests, guidance on sexuality and sexually transmitted diseases were also mentioned.

The research made it possible to find out about the situations that facilitate working with women, which are the establishment of a bond, the presence of community health agents, the gender issue, the audience of mature women, the organisation of the service in the unit, the good relationship between the team and improvements in the Women's Health room. It also revealed the situations that prevail as hindering the work: the lack of materials and financial resources, difficulty in women's access to the ESF units, low attendance by women at preventive examinations, lack of support from management and administrators, the unit's opening hours being incompatible for working women, women's participation in the groups, the types of contraceptives offered to women, nomadic families, care for areas without territory or health agents and the lack of medication (folic acid).

The main strategies used at work to address women's health include: active search, group care, follow-up, involvement, partnerships with universities, facilitating access to the service, team meetings, leaving the door open to the service whenever necessary and a waiting room.

The team meeting is considered by the nurses to be a fundamental occasion for strategic decisions for the work, learning, exchange of knowledge and ideas, and the active search for and follow-up of women takes place through a synchronised partnership with the health agents.

As for continuing education activities, the nurses say that they receive regular training in various areas and that women's health is often on the agenda.

The results show that the nurses' work with women is based on the norms and protocols established by the Ministry of Health, with the aim of promoting, preventing and controlling health problems. However, the nurses emphasise that the work could focus less on routine practices and place more value on actions geared towards the cultural and economic context, listening, bonding, welcoming, the needs of the users and co-responsibility for care. Therefore, the work of caring for women requires the involvement of all the professionals in the Family Health Team, as well as the mobilisation of management to make it possible to devise new actions and quality services for users of the Unified Health System.

The conclusion is that the ESF units are great spaces for professional training and empowerment of constitutional rights, and that the health team is also the basis for their success or otherwise, since it is this team that seeks out, keeps or alienates the community in its area, depending on the strategies used and whether they meet the population's wishes.

From this study, we hope to help ensure that nurses' work with women in the ESF units in Santa Maria is recognised by managers and health professionals for their efforts to carry out their work based on the standards and protocols established by the Ministry of Health, with the aim of promoting, preventing and controlling health problems; to constantly seek strategies to overcome the difficulties that arise at work, and to use technologies to help organise the work process. As a result, new actions and new quality services for users of the Unified Health System can be made possible and idealised.

The difficulty encountered during the study was scheduling interviews with nurses, as they have many duties which limit their time. The limitations were the specific nature of the subject and the scarcity of studies on the same subject, which made it necessary to draw some conclusions from research on nurses' work with the elderly, men and children.

In this sense, it is suggested that further studies be carried out to find out more about the work process of FHS teams, in order to better characterise the work of nurses in FHS units.

CHAPTER 6

REFERENCES

ARAÚJO, M. B. S.; ROCHA, P. M. Teamwork: a challenge for the consolidation of the family health strategy. **Revista Ciência & Saúde coletiva**, Rio de Janeiro, v. 12, n. 2, p. 455-464, 2007. Available at: < http://www.redalyc.org/pdf/630/63012219.pdf>. Accessed on: 21 August 2012.

ARAÚJO, M. F. S. The nurse in the Family Health Programme: professional practice and identity construction. **Revista Conceitos,** p. 39-43, 2005. Available at: < http://www.saude.ms.gov.br/controle/ShowFile.php?id=53553>. Accessed on: 21 August 2013.

ARANTES, C. I. S. et al. O Controle Social no Sistema Único de Saúde: Concepções e Ações e Enfermeiras da Atenção Básica. **Revista Texto Contexto Enfermagem**, Florianópolis, v. 16, n. 3, p. 470-478, jul./set. 2007. Available at: < http://www.scielo.br/pdf/tce/vl6n3/al3vl6n3.pdf>. Accessed on: 16 Sep. 2013.

BRAZIL. Law n. 7.498, of 25 June 1986. Provides for the regulation of nursing practice and makes other provisions. **Official Gazette of the Federative Republic of Brazil,** Brasília, DF, 25 June 1986. Available at: < http://www.planalto.gov.br/ccivil_03/leis/L7498.htm>. Accessed on: 16 Nov. 2013.

. Law n. 8.080, of 19 September 1990. Provides for the conditions for the promotion, protection and recovery of health, the organisation and operation of the corresponding services and makes other provisions. **Official Gazette of the Federative Republic of Brazil,** Brasília, DF, 20 September 1990a. Available at: < http://www.planalto.gov.br/ccivil_03/leis/18080.htm>. Accessed on: 16 Nov. 2012.

______. Law No. 8.142, of 28 December 1990. Provides for community participation in the management of the Unified Health System (SUS) and intergovernmental transfers of financial resources in the health area, and makes other provisions. **Official Gazette of the Federative Republic of Brazil,** Brasília, DF, 28 Dec. 1990b. Available at: < http://www.planalto.gov.br/ccivil_03/leis/18142.htm>. Accessed on: 16 Nov. 2012.

. Ministry of Health. Health Care Secretariat. Coordination of Community Health. **Saúde da Família:** uma estratégia para a reorientação do modelo assistencial. Brasília: Ministry of Health, 1997. Available at: <http://bvsms.saude.gov.br/bvs/publicacoes/cd09_16.pdf>. Accessed on: 10 Nov. 2012.

. Ministry of Health. Executive Secretariat. **Family Health Programme.** Brasília:

Ministry of Health, 2001a. Available at: <http://www.ccms.saude.gov.br/saudebateaporta/mostravirtual/publicacoes/psf01.pdf >. Accessed on: 9 Nov. 2012.

. Ministry of Health. Secretary of Public Policy. **Practical Guide to the Family Health Programme.** Brasília: Ministry of Health, 2001b. Part 1. Available at: < http://189.28.128.100/dab/docs/publicacoes/geral/guia_pratico_sau de_familia_psfl .pdf>. Accessed on: 10 Nov. 2012.

. Ministry of Health. Secretary of Public Policy. **Practical Guide to the Family Health Programme.** Brasília: Ministry of Health, 2001c. Part 2. Available at: <http://l89.28.128.100/dab/docs/publicacoes/geral/guia_pratico_saud e_familia_psf2.pdf>. Accessed on: 10 Nov. 2012.

. Ministry of Health. The role of nurses in primary care. **Informe da Atenção Básica.** n° 16, ano III, abril de 2002a. Available at: < http://189.28.128.10 0/dab/docs/publicacoes/informes/psfinfol6.pdf>. Accessed on: 9 Nov. 2012.

. Ministry of Health. Secretariat for Health Policies. Women's Health Technical Area. **Family Planning Assistance:** Technical Manual. 4. ed. Brasília: Ministry of Health, 2002b. Available at: < http://bvsms.saude.gov.br/bvs /publicacoes/0102assistencial.pdf>. Accessed on: 9 Nov. 2012.

. Ministry of Health. Executive Secretariat. **HumanizaSUS:** national humanisation policy: basic document for SUS managers and workers. 1. ed. Brasília: Ministry of Health, 2004. Available at: < http://bvsms.saude.gov.br/bvs/ publicacoes/humanizaSus_doc_base.pdf>. Accessed on: 9 Nov. 2013.

. GM Ordinance No. 648, of 28 March 2006. Approves the National Primary Care Policy, establishing revised guidelines and norms for the organisation of Primary Care for the Family Health Programme (PSF) and the Community Health Agents Programme (PACS). **Official Gazette of the Federative Republic of Brazil,** Brasília, DF, 28 March 2006a. Available at: <http://www.brasilsus.com.br/le gislacoes/gm/899-648.html?q=portaria>. Accessed on: 16 Nov. 2012.

. Ministry of Health. Health Care Secretariat. Department of Strategic Programme Actions. **Prenatal and postpartum** care: qualified and humanised care - Technical manual. 3.ed. Brasília: Ministry of Health, 2006b. Available at: < http://portal.saude.gov.br/portal/arquivos/pdfimanual_puerperio_2006.pdf>. Accessed on: 9 Nov. 2012.

. Ministry of Health. Health Care Secretariat. Department of Primary Care. **Control of cervical and breast cancers.** 1. ed. Brasília: Ministry of Health, 2006c. Available at: < http://portal.saude.gov.br/port al/arquivos/pdficademo_atencao_basica.pdf>. Accessed on: 9 Nov. 2012.

. GM Ordinance No. 154, of 24 January 2008. Creates the Family Health Support Centres (NASF). **Official Gazette of the Federative Republic of Brazil,** Brasília, DF, 25 January 2008. Available at: <http://189.28.128.100/dab/docs/legislaca o/portarial54_24_01_08.pdf>. Accessed on: 12 Nov. 2012.

. Ministry of Health. **Special:** Health guarantees more protection for women. 2009a. Available at: < http://portal.saude.gov.br/portal/aplicacoes/reportagensEspe ciais/default.cfm?pg=dspDetalhes&id_area= 124&CO_NOTICIA=10007>. Accessed on: 10 September 2012.

. Portal Brasil. **Saúde:** SUS democratises citizens' access to health services. 2009b. Available at: < http://www.brasil.gov.br/saude/2009/ll/sus- democratiza-o-acesso-do-cidadao-a aos-servicos-de-saude>. Accessed on: 04 October 2013.

. Resolution number 358, of 15 October 2009. Provides for the Systematisation of Nursing Care and the implementation of the Nursing Process in public or private environments where professional nursing care takes place, and makes other provisions. Federal Nursing Council. Brasília, 2009c. Available at: < http://novo.portalcofen.gov.br/resolu o-cofen-3582009_4384.html>. Accessed on: 18 Nov. 2013.

. National Council of Health Secretaries. **Primary Care and Health Promotion.** National Council of Health Secretaries. Brasília: CONASS, 2011a. Available at:< http://www.conass.org.br/colecao2011/livro_3.pdf>. Accessed on: 28 Nov. 2012.

. Ministry of Health. Health Care Secretariat. Department of Strategic Programme Actions. **National Policy for Comprehensive Women's Health Care:** Principles and Guidelines. 1. ed., 2. reimpr. Brasília: Ministry of Health, 2011b. Available at: <http://bvsms.saude.gov.br/bvs/publicacoes/politica_naciona_ mulher_principios_diretrizes.pdf>. Accessed on: 9 Nov. 2012.

. Blog do Planalto. **Stork Network will provide care for women from pregnancy to the baby's second year.** Blog do Planalto, 28 March 2011c. Available at: <http://blog.planalto.gov.br/rede-cegonha-dara-atendimento-a-mulher-da-gravidezate -o-segundo-ano-do-be/>. Accessed on: 22 Feb. 2013.

. Ministry of Health. Health Care Secretariat. Primary Care Department. **Welcoming spontaneous demand.** 1. ed. Brasília: Ministry of Health, 201 ld. Available at: <http://189.28.128.100/dab/docs/publicacoes/geral/miolo_CA P_28.pdf>. Accessed on: 22 Feb. 2013.

. Ministry of Health. Health Care Secretariat. Department of Primary Care. **National Primary Care Policy.** 1. ed. Brasília: Ministry of Health, 2012a. Available at: < http://189.28.128.100/dab/docs/publicacoes/geral/pn ab.pdf>. Accessed on: 12 Nov. 2012.

. **Resolution number 466,** of 12 December 2012. Provides for guidelines and regulatory standards for research involving human beings. National Health Council. Brasília, 2012b. Available at: < http://conselho.saude .gov.br/resolucoes/2012/Reso466.pdf>. Accessed on: 18 Nov. 2013.

. Ministry of Health. Health Portal. **Accompanying mother in labour brings more safety to the mother.** Brasília, 2013a. Available at: <http://portal.saude.gov.br/p ortal/saude/visualizar_texto.cfm?idtxt=24112>. Accessed on: 30 May 2012.

. Ministry of Health. Health Portal. **Women's Health.** Brasília, 2013b. Available at: <http://portal.saude.gov.br/portal/saude/visualizar_texto.cfin?idtxt=2 5236>. Accessed on: 9 Nov. 2012.

. Ministry of Health. Health Portal. **Stork Network.** Brasília, 2013c. Available at: <http://portal.saude.gov.br/PORTAL/SAUDE/GESTOR/AREA.CFM ?ID_AREA=1816>. Accessed on: 22 Feb. 2013.

CAGNIN, E. R. G. **Nursing care for women in the pregnancy-puerperium cycle:** the reality of Araraquara/SP. 2008. 158 f. Dissertation (Master's in Public Health Nursing) - University of São Paulo, Ribeirão Preto, 2008. Available at: <http://www.teses.usp.br/teses/disponiveis/22/22133/tde-06032009- O8513.php>. Accessed on: 24 September 2012.

CAMPOS, G. W. S. **Reforma da reforma:** repensando a saúde. 3. ed. São Paulo: Hucitec, 2006.

COELHO, M. O.; JORGE, M. S. B. Tecnologia das relações como dispositivo do atendimento humanizada na atenção básica à saúde na perspectiva do acesso, do acolhimento e do vínculo. **Revista Ciência & Saúde Coletiva,** v. 14, supl. 1, p. 1523-1531, 2009. Available at: < http://www.scielo.br/pdi7csc/vl4sl/a26vl4sl.pdf >. Accessed: 23 August 2013.

CORREIA, M. V. C. **Que controle social:** os conselhos de saúde como instrumento. 2. ed. Rio de Janeiro: Fiocruz, 2000.

COSTA, F. B. da; TRINDADE, M. A. do N.; PEREIRA, M. L. A Inserção do Biomédico no Programa de Saúde da Família. **Revista Eletrónica Novo Enfoque,** v. 11, n. 11, p. 27-33, 2010. Available at: < http://www.castelobranco.br/sistema/nov oenfoque/files/1 l/artigos/04.pdf>. Accessed on: 12 Nov. 2012.

COSTA, P. et al. Comprehensive Women's Health Care: Reflecting on Public Policies. In: 3ª JORNADA INTERDISCIPLINAR EM SAÚDE, 4., 2010, Santa Maria. **Proceedings...** Santa Maria: Unifra, 2010. Available at: < http://www.unifra.br/ev entos/jis2010/Trabalhos/263.pdf>. Accessed: 9 August 2012.

CUNHA, A. F. et al. Actions to promote women's health: an experience report. **Revista UDESC em Ação,** v. 5, n. 1, 2011. Available at: <http://www.revistas.udesc.br/index.php/udescemacao/article/view/2237/pdf_72>. Accessed on: 20 May 2012.

CUNHA, S. M. B. et al. Organisation of Nursing Work in Family Health Strategies in the Municipality of Cáceres-MT. **Revista Eletrónica Gestão & Saúde,** v. 4, n. 2, 2013. Available at: <http://gestaoesaude.unb.br/index.php/gestaoesaude/article/view/491/pdf>. Accessed on: 21 May 2012.

DATASUS. **Health Information Booklet.** 2012. Available at: <http://tabnet.datasus.gov.br/cgi/tabcgi.exe7ibge/cnv/poprs.def>. Accessed on: 9 August 2012.

ERMEL, R. C.; FRACOLLI, L. A. The work of nurses in the Family Health Programme in Marília/SP. **Revista Escola de Enfermagem USP,** v. 40, n. 4, p. 533-539, 2006. Available at: <http://www.ee.usp.br/reeusp/upload/pdf/286.pdf>. Accessed on: 13 March 2012.

FACCFUNI, L. A. et al. Performance of the PSF in the South and Northeast of Brazil: institutional and epidemiological evaluation of Primary Health Care. **Journal Ciência & Saúde Coletiva,** v. 11, n. 3, p. 669-681, 2006. Available at: <http://www.scielo.br/pdf/csc /vl ln3/30982.pdf>. Accessed on: 12 March 2012.

FELLI, V. E. A.; PEDUZZI, M. Managerial work in nursing. In: KURGANT, P. et al. **Management in nursing.** Rio de Janeiro: Guanabara Koogan, 2005. p. 1-13.

FRANCO, T. B.; MERHY, E. E. Family Health Programme (PSF): Contradictions of a Programme aimed at changing the techno-assistance model. In: MERHY, E. E. et al. (Orgs.). **O trabalho em saúde:** olhando e experienciando o SUS no cotidiano. 4. ed. São Paulo: Hucitec, 2007.

FRANCO, B. T.; BUENO, W. S.; MERHY, E. E. O acolhimento e os processos de trabalho em saúde: o caso Betim MG. In: MERHY, E. E. et al. (Orgs.). **Health work:** looking at and experiencing the SUS in everyday life. 4. ed. São Paulo: Hucitec, 2007.

FREITAS, M. C. M. C.; NUNES, B. M. V. T. O processo de trabalho do enfermeiro na Estratégia da Saúde da Família. **Revista Interdisciplinar NOVAFAPI**, Teresina, v. 3, n. 3, p. 39-43, jul./set. 2010. Available at:<http://www.novafapi.com.br/sistemas/revistainterdisciplinar/pdf/revistavol3n3.pdf>. Accessed on: 23 September 2012.

GIL, A. **C. Como elaborar projetos de pesquisa.** 5. ed. São Paulo: Atlas, 2010.

GOMES, L. O. S. **Work Process in the Family Health Programme:** From the Health Team's Perspective. 2011. 200 f. Dissertation (Master's in Nursing and Health)-State

University of Southwest Bahia, Jequié, 2011. Available at: < http://www.uesb.br/ppgenfsaude/dissertacoes/turma2/DISSERTACAO-LIANE-OLI VEIRA-SOUZA-GOMES.pdf>. Accessed on: 06 Sep. 2013.

HORTA et al. The Practice of Groups as a Health Promotion Action in the Family Health Strategy. **Revista APS:** Atenção Primária à Saúde, Juiz de Fora, v. 12, n. 3, p. 293-301, jul./set. 2009. Available at: < http://www.seer.ufjf.br/index.php/aps/arti cle/viewFile/407/228>. Accessed on: 26 August 2013.

LEOPARDI, M. T. **Metodologia da pesquisa na saúde.** Santa Maria (RS): Pallotti, 2001.

LEONELLO, V. M.; OLIVEIRA, M. A. C. Competences for the nurse's educational action. **Revista Latino-Americana de Enfermagem** *[oniine],* v. 16, n. 2, p. 177-183. 2008. Available at: <http://www.scielo.br/pdf/rlae/vl6n2/pt_02.pdf>. Accessed on: 29 August 2013.

LOPES, M. C. L.; MARCON, S. S. Family care in primary care: facilities and difficulties faced by health professionals. **Acta Scientiarum.** Health Science, Maringá, v. 34, n. 1, p. 85-93, jan./jun. 2012. Available at: <http://www.periodicos.uem.br/oj s/index.php/ActaSciHealthSci/articl e/view/7624/pdf>. Accessed on: 23 October 2013.

MADEIRA, K. H. **Interdisciplinary Work Practices in Family Health:** a case study. 2009. 148f. Dissertation (Master's Degree in Health and Labour Management) - Universidade do Vale do Itajaí, Itajaí, 2009. Available at: < http://www6.univali.br/tede/tde_arquivos/4/TDE-2009-08-10T091148Z-503/Publico/ Karin%20Hamerski%20Madeira.pdf>. Accessed on: 23 October 2013.

MATTA, G. C.; MOROSINI, M. V. G. Primary Health Care. In: PEREIRA, I. B.; LIMA, J. C. F. **Dicionário da Educação Profissional em Saúde.** 2. ed. rev. ampl. Rio de Janeiro: EPSJV, 2008. Available at: <http:// www.epsjv.fiocruz.br/dicionario/verbete/atepri sau.html>. Accessed on: 23 October 2013.

MATTOS, E.; PIRES, D. E. P. de.; CAMPOS, W. de S. Work relationships in interdisciplinary teams: contributions to the constitution of new forms of health work organisation. **Brazilian Journal of Nursing.** Brasília, v. 62, n. 6, p. 863-869, nov./dez. 2009. Available at:< http://www.scielo.br/scielo.php ?script=sci_arttext&pid=S0034-71672009000600010&lng=en&nrm=iso&tlng=en>. Accessed on: 23 October 2013.

MATUMOTO, S.; MISHIMA, S. M.; PINTO, I. C. Collective Health: a challenge for nursing. **Caderno Saúde Pública.** Rio de Janeiro, v. 17, n. 1, p. 233-241, jan./feb. 2001. Available at: < http://www.scielo.br/pdf/csp/vl7nl/4080.pdf>. Accessed on: 23 October 2013.

MENDES, E. V. **Primary Health Care in the SUS.** Fortaleza: Ceará School of Public Health, 2002.

MENDES-GONÇALVES, R. B. **Tecnologia e Organização Social das Práticas de Saúde:** características tecnológicas de processo de trabalho na rede estadual de centros de saúde de São Paulo. São Paulo: Hucitec, 1994.

MERHY, E. E. In search of quality in health services: open-door health services and the techno-assistance model in defence of life. In: Cecílio L.C.O, (Org.). **Inventing change in health.** São Paulo: Hucitec; 1994. p. 116-160.

. **Saúde:** a cartografia do Trabalho Vivo. São Paulo: Hucitec, 2002.

. et al (Orgs.). **Health Work:** looking at and experiencing the SUS in everyday life. São Paulo: Hucitec, 2003.

. In search of lost time: the micropolitics of living labour in health. In: MERHY, E. E.; ONOCKO, R. (Orgs.). **Acting in health:** a challenge for the public. 3 ed. São Paulo: Hucitec, 2007. p. 71-112.

MINAYO, M. C. S. **O desafio do Conhecimento.** Qualitative research in health. 12. ed. São Paulo: Hucitec, 2010.

MIRANDA, R. M. de. **Importância do Grupo operativo na Melhoria da Assistência a Gestante na Estratégia Saúde da Família.** 2011. 38f. Monograph (Specialisation in Primary Care in Family Health) - Federal University of Minas Gerais, Belo Horizonte, 2011. Available at: < http://www.nescon.medicina.ufing.br/biblioteca/imagem/3010.pdf>. Accessed: 02 September 2013.

MONTENEGRO, L. C. **The Professional Training of Nurses: Advances and Challenges for their Performance in Primary Health Care.** 2010. 98 f. Dissertation (Master's Degree in Nursing) - Federal University of Minas Gerais, Belo Horizonte, 2010. Available at: <http://www.bibliotecadigital.ufing.br/dspace/handle/1843/GCPA-84RHCD>. Accessed on: 07 October 2013.

MUNARI, D. B. et al. Contributions to the psychological dimension of groups. **Revista Enfermagem UERJ.** Rio de Janeiro, v.15, n. 1, p. 107-112, 2007. Available at: < http://www.revenf.bvs.br/pdfireuerj/vl5nl/vl5nlal7.pdf>. Accessed on: 30 October 2013.

OLIVEIRA, C. L. et al. An experience of women's empowerment in Primary Health Care. **Brazilian Journal of Family and Community Medicine.** Florianópolis, v. 6, n. 21, p. 283-287, Oct./Dec. 2011. Available at:< http://www.rbmfc.org.br/index.php/rbmfc/article/view/325/387>. Accessed on: 30 October 2013.

PASSOS, C. M. dos. **The work of nurses in primary care in Belo Horizonte:** Evaluation of programme actions. 2011. 119 f. Dissertation (Master's in Nursing) - Federal University of Minas Gerais, Belo Horizonte, 2011. Available at:< http://www.enf.ufing.br/site_novo/modules/mastop_publish/files/fil es_4dca78ff63bc4.pdf>. Accessed on: 09 August 2012.

PEDUZZI, M. **Multiprofessional health team:** the interface between work and interaction. 1998. 254f. Thesis (Doctorate) - Faculty of Medical Sciences, State University of Campinas, Campinas, 1998. Available at:< http://www.a cervo.epsjv.fiocruz.br/beb/textocompleto/003744>. Accessed on: 09 August 2012.

PEDUZZI, M.; ALSEMI, M. L. O processo de enfermagem: a cisão entre planejamento e execução do cuidado. **Revista Brasileira de Enfermagem,** Brasília, v. 55, n. 4, p. 392-398, Jul./Aug. 2002. Available at: < http://bvsms.saude.gov.br/bvs/is_digital/is_0303/pdfs/IS23(3)066.pdf>. Accessed on: 21 September 2012.

PINHEIRO, G. M. L. **Nursing Work Process in Elderly Care within the Family Health Strategy.** 2011. 169f. Thesis (Doctorate) - Federal University of Santa Catarina, Florianópolis, 2011. Available at: <http://repositorio.ufsc.br/xmlui/bitstream/handle/123456789/95573/291990.pdf/seq uence=l>. Accessed on: 16 Nov. 2012.

PINTO, E. S. G. **Difficulties and/or facilities experienced by Family Health Strategy professionals.** 2008. 119 f. Dissertation (Master's in Nursing) - Federal University of Rio Grande do Norte, Natal, 2008. Available at:< http://www.natal.rn.gov.br/bvn/publicacoes/erikasgp.pdf>. Accessed on: 18 October 2013.

PIRES, D. **Reestruturação produtiva e trabalho em saúde no Brasil.** 2 ed. Pinheiros: Anablume, 2008.

RAMOS, C. S. et al. Profile of nurses working in the family health strategy. **Revista Ciência, Cuidado e Saúde,** v. 8, suplem. p. 85-91, 2009. Available at: < http://periodicos.uem.br/ojs/index.php/CiencCuidSaude/article/view/9722/5535>. Accessed on: 12 March 2012.

ROCHA, S. M. M.; ALMEIDA, M. C. P. de. The nursing work process in collective health and interdisciplinarity. **Latin American Journal of**

Enfermagem, Ribeirão Preto, v. 8, n. 6, p. 96-101, dec./2000. Available at: < http://www. scielo. br/pdf/rlae/v8n6/12354.pdf>. Accessed on: 26 April 2012.

ROSA, W. A. G.; LABATE, R. C. Family health programme: Building a new model of care. **Revista Latino-Americana de Enfermagem**, Ribeirão Preto, v.13, n. 6, p.

1027-1034, 2005. Available at: < http://www.scielo.br/pdf/rlae/ vl3n6/vl3n6al6.pdf>. Accessed on: 26 April 2012.

SALMERON, N. A.; FUCÍTALO, A. R. Programa de Saúde de Família: O papel do enfermeiro na área da Saúde da Mulher. **Revista Saúde Coletiva,** São Paulo, v. 4, n. 19, p. 25-29, 2008. Available at: < http://www.redalyc.org/redalyc/pdf/842/842019 O6.pdf>. Accessed on: 14 August 2012.

SANNA, M. C. Nursing work processes. **Revista Brasileira de Enfermagem,** Brasília, v. 60, n. 2, p. 221-224, Mar./Apr. 2007. Available at: < http://www.scielo.br/pdf/reben/v60n2/al7v60n2.pdP>. Accessed on: 26 Apr. 2012.

SANTANA, J. C. B. et al. Community Health Agent: Perceptions in the Family Health Strategy. **Revista Cogitare Enfermagem.** Paraná, v. 14, n. 4, p. 645-652, Oct./Dec. 2009. Available at: <http://ojs.c3sl.ufpr.br/ojs2/index.php/cogitare/article/ view/16377/10858>. Accessed on: 30 October 2013.

SANTOS, B. R. dos. **The Family Health Strategy and adolescent care.** 2011.176 f. Dissertation (Master's in Psychology) - Federal University of Santa Maria, Santa Maria, 2011. Available at: <http://cascavel.cpd.ufsm.br/tede/tde_arquivos/41/TDE-2011-04-05T163701Z-3109/ Publico/SANTOS,%20BIBIANA%20RAMOS%20DOS.pdf>. Accessed on: 12 Nov. 2012.

SANTOS, E. M.; MORAIS, S. H. G. Home Visits in the Family Health Strategy: nurses' perceptions. **Revista Cogitare Enfermagem,** v. 16, n. 3, p. 492-497, 2011. Available at: < http://ojs.c3sl.ufpr.br/ojs2/index.php/cogitare/article /view/21761/16235>. Accessed on: 13 Mar.12.

SANTOS, V. C.; SOARES, C. B.; CAMPOS, C. M. S. A relação trabalho-saúde de enfermeiros do PSF no município de São Paulo. **Revista Escola de Enfermagem USP,** v. 41, Esp., p. 777-781, 2007. Available at:<http://www.scielo.br/pdf/reeusp/ v41nspe/v41nspea05.pdf>. Accessed on: 13 March 2012.

SCFUMITH, M. D.; LIMA, M. A. D. S. The nurse in the Family Health Team: a case study. **Revista Enfermagem UERJ,** v. 17, n. 2, p. 252-256, 2009. Available at: <http://www.facenf.uerj.br/vl7n2/vl7n2a20.pdf>. Accessed on: 12 Mar.12.

SEVERINO, J. G.; COSTA, N. C. G. Atuação do enfermeiro no atendimento à mulher na saúde da família em Diamantino, Mato Grosso. **Revista Matogrossense de Enfermagem,** Mato Grosso, v. 1, n. 2, p. 166-182, nov./dez. 2010. Available at:<http://www.portaldeperiodicos.uned.edu.br/index.php/REMENFE/article/view/4 33/305>. Accessed on: 10 August 2012.

SILVA, C. P.; MARTINS, M. C. M. Nursing work process in the Family Health

Strategy: dilemmas and perspectives. **SANARE - Revista de Políticas Públicas,** v. 8, n. 2, p. 91-101, jul./dez. 2009. Available at: <http://sanare.emnuvens.com.br/sanare/article/view/23/19>. Accessed on: 13 March 2012.

TAVARES, L. F. The evolution of work and the human being. **The Administration Portal.** 2011. Available at: <http://www.administradores.com.br/informe-se/artigos/a-evolucao-do-trabalho-e-o-ser-humano/55179/>. Accessed on: 10 October 2012.

VASCONCELOS, M.; GRILLO, M. J. C.; SOARES, S. M. **Pedagogical Practices in Primary Health Care.** Technologies for approaching the individual, family and community. Belo Horizonte: UFMG. 2009. Available at: https://ares.unasus.gov.br/acervo/handle/ARES/93>. Accessed on: 02 September 2013.

ZAGONEL, I. P. S. Nursing consultation: a model of methodology for care. In: CARRARO, T. E.; WESTPHALEN, M. E. A. (Orgs.). **Methodologies for Nursing Care:** theorising, models and subsidies for practice. 1. ed. Goiânia: AB, 2001.

APPENDICES

Appendix A - Interview script with nurses

FEDERAL UNIVERSITY OF SANTA MARIA HEALTH SCIENCES CENTRE POSTGRADUATE NURSING PROGRAMME INTERVIEW SCRIPT

Research:^{U} **Nurses' work with women in the Family Health Strategy".**

PERSONAL AND PROFESSIONAL IDENTITY

DATE: .... Identification Code: E:..................

1. Identification Data:

1.1 Year of Birth: []

1.2 Sex: [1] Male [2] Female

2. Professional training data

2.1 Year Graduated: []

2.2 Nature of Institution: [1] Public [2] Private UF: []

2.3 Do you have another degree: [1] Yes [2] No

2.4 [1] Health [2] Other areas Which?

1.5 Postgraduate Lato Sensu: [1] Yes [2] No

1.5.1 Area: Year

conclusion: []

1.5.2 Area: Year

conclusion: []

[5] other ....

1.6 Stricto Sensu Postgraduate Programme:

1.6.1 Master's degree: [1] Yes [2] No

1.6.2 Area: Year

conclusion: []

1.6.3 Doctorate: [1] Yes [2] No

1.6.4 Area: Year

conclusion: []

1.7 Have you taken part in training? [1] Yes [2] No

1.7.1 Area: ____

1.7.2 Area: ____

1.7.3 Area: ____

1.8 How often do you take part in these trainings? [1] annually [2] twice a year

[3] more than twice a year .... [4] monthly

[5] other ....

1.9 What was the date of your last training course? Month/Year: [*I]*

4. Data on professional relationships:

5. ABOUT THE WORK

5.1 Time working in nursing [1] 1 to 5 years ....[2] 6 to 10 years
[3] 11 to 15 years..[4] 16 years and over
[5] other ....

5.2 Time working in the Family Health Strategy [1] 1 to 5 years [2] 6 to 10 years
[3] 11 to 15 years..[4] 16 years and over
[5] other ....

Open questions:

1 How is the care of women organised in this FHS unit?

2 What actions does the nurse carry out with women in the ESF unit?

3 What facilities and difficulties do you find in carrying out actions with women in the FHS unit?

4 What strategies do you use to deal with these facilities/difficulties in your work with women in the ESF Unit?

5 Which professionals on the team are involved in working with women in what way?

óWould you have any suggestions for improving the work with women in the ESF units? What are they?

Appendix B - Informed Consent Form

FEDERAL UNIVERSITY OF SANTA MARIA HEALTH SCIENCES CENTRE POSTGRADUATE PROGRAMME IN NURSING

Study title: Nurses' work with women in the Family Health Strategy

Researcher responsible: Suzinara Beatriz Soares de Lima

Master's student researcher: Nurse Francislene Lopes Menezes
Institution/Department: Federal University of Santa Maria / Course of Postgraduate Diploma in Nursing

Contact telephone number: (55) 3220-8263

Data collection site: Family Health Strategies in Santa Maria/RS

INFORMED CONSENT FORM

Dear Sir or Madam,

You are being invited to answer the questions in this questionnaire on a completely voluntary basis. Before you agree to take part in this research and answer this questionnaire, it is very important that you understand the information and instructions contained in this document. The researchers should answer all your questions before you decide to take part. You have the right to withdraw from participating in the research at any time, without any penalty and without losing the benefits to which you are entitled.

The aims of the study are: to find out how nurses work with women in the Family Health Strategy (FHS) units in the municipality of Santa Maria/RS; to identify the facilities and difficulties of nurses' work with women in the FHS units; to identify the strategies used by nurses when working with women in the FHS units; and to analyse nurses' work with women in the FHS units.

Your participation in this research will take the form of an individual interview, which will be recorded on MP3 audio, in which the researcher will ask you a few questions. If you do not wish to be recorded, your wishes will be respected and this will not make the interview unfeasible, as the researcher will take note of your account.

Interviews must be scheduled in advance according to the interviewee's availability. What you say will be typed up (transcribed) and the recordings will be kept for five years, as determined by the ethics of the research, after which time they will be destroyed. Only the researchers involved in this research will have access to the recordings.

The information you provide will contribute to increasing knowledge in health and nursing, as well as to further research on this subject.

In principle, the study does not foresee any kind of risk to the research subjects, and if any kind of emotional discomfort arises due to a memory, I will be able to conclude the interview and refer you to a professional in the service who has been previously agreed upon.

At the end of this research, the results will be published in the form of a dissertation and articles in scientific nursing journals. The privacy of the information you provide will be guaranteed by the researchers responsible. The research subjects will not be identified at any time. They will be identified by the initial letter E (El, E2, E3, E4...) of the word Nurse. The written information will be kept under the responsibility of Enf* Profi Dr[3] Suzinara Beatriz Soares de Lima (supervisor of this research), in her personal, locked cupboard, in room 1304B, at the Health Sciences Centre of the Federal University of Santa Maria (UFSM), for five years, after which time it will be destroyed.

I am aware of and agree ________________________ to participate in this research by signing this consent form in two copies, keeping one of them.

Santa Maria, from 20

Participant's signature Signature of researcher

If you have any concerns or questions about the ethics of the research, please contact: Research Ethics Committee - UFSM - Cidade Universitária - Bairro Camobi, Av. Roraima, n°1000 - CEP: 97.105.900 Santa Maria - RS. Telephone: (55) 3220-9362 - Fax: (55)3220-8009 Email: comiteeticapesquisa@smail.ufsm.br. Web: www.ufsm.br/cep

Appendix C - Confidentiality Agreement

CONFIDENTIALITY AGREEMENT

Research title: Nurses' work with women in the Family Health Strategy

Author: Nun. Mda. Francislene Lopes Menezes

Supervisor/Researcher: Prof **Dr Suzinara Beatriz** Soares Lima. Dr Suzinara Beatriz Soares de Lima.

The researchers of this project undertake to preserve the privacy of the nurses who take part in the research, whose data will be collected by means of semi-structured interviews, using audio recording and carried out in the workplace, at a time agreed with the participants. They also agree that this information will be used solely and exclusively to carry out this project, to build a database for the Nursing and Health Management Group, which is linked to the Care, Health and Nursing Research Group of the UFSM Nursing Department, and to develop the research. The information may only be disclosed anonymously and will be kept for a period of five years under the responsibility of Suzinara Beatriz Soares de Lima (supervisor of this research), in her personal locked cabinet in room 1304B at the Health Sciences Centre - UFSM, after which time the data will be destroyed. This research project was reviewed and approved by the Research Ethics Committee of UFSM on ....// , with the number of

CAAE ....

Santa Maria, ... from .... 20..........

Francislenc L. Menezes
REGISTRATION:
201260761
COREN: 221.363

Suzinara Beatriz S. de Lima
SIAPE: 2100943
COREN: 56571

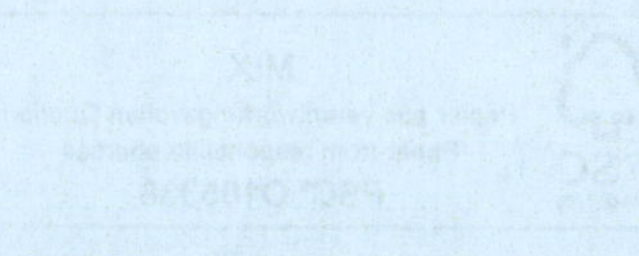

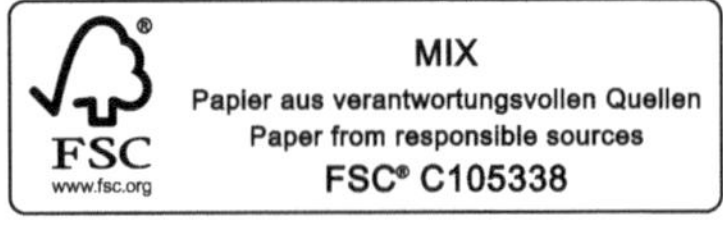

Printed by Books on Demand GmbH, Norderstedt / Germany